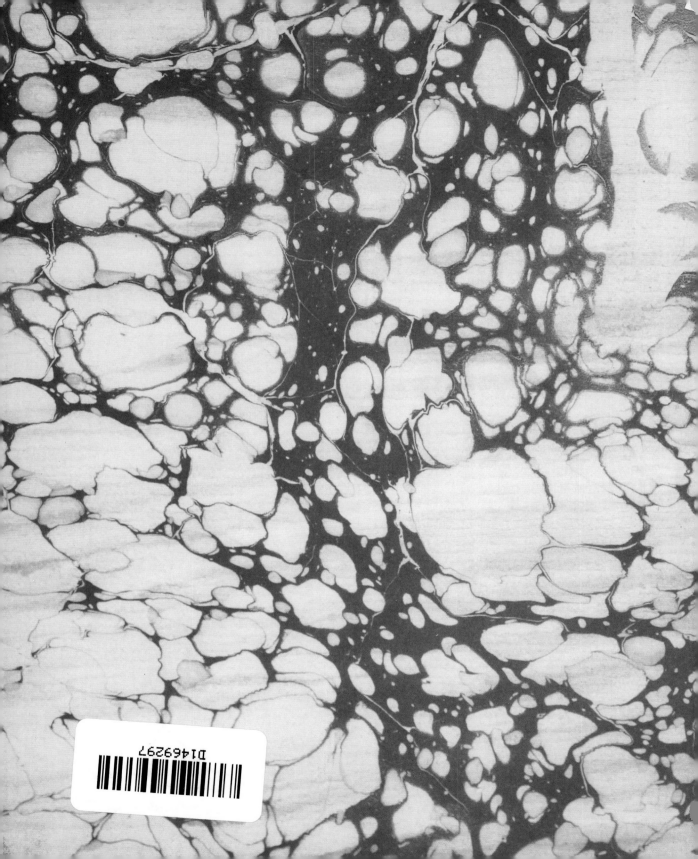

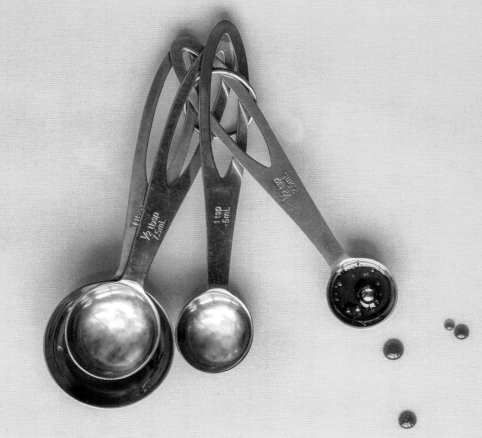

THE CBD KITCHEN

THE
CBD KITCHEN

Over 50 plant-based recipes
for tonics, easy meals, treats
& skincare made with the
goodness extracted from hemp

LEAH VANDERVELDT
Photography by Clare Winfield

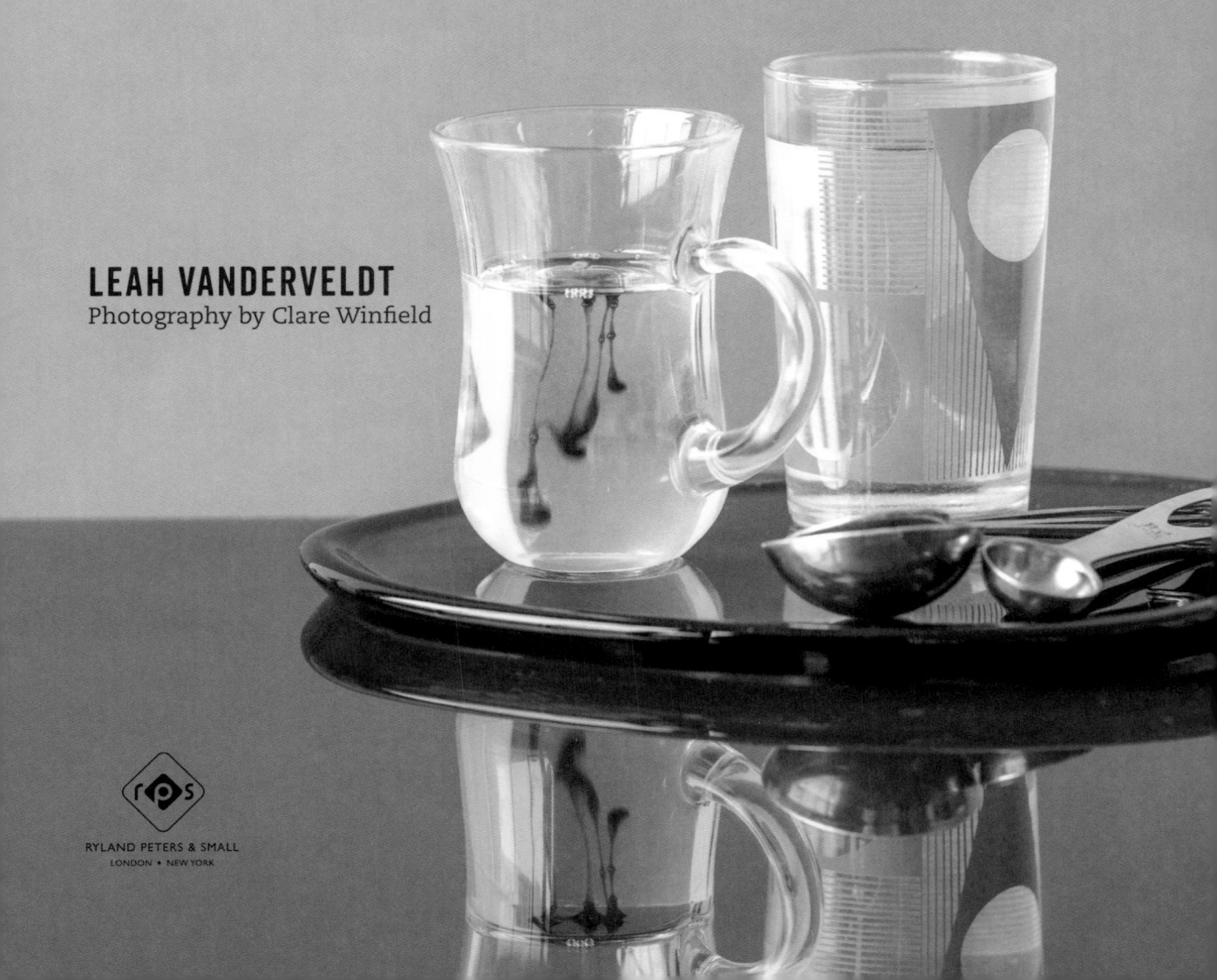

rps
RYLAND PETERS & SMALL
LONDON • NEW YORK

Dedication

For anyone seeking better health and more calm in their lives.

Senior designer Megan Smith
Commissioning editor
  Alice Sambrook
Head of production
  Patricia Harrington
Art director Leslie Harrington
Editorial director Julia Charles
Publisher Cindy Richards

Prop stylist Alexander Breeze
Food stylist Maud Eden
Indexer Vanessa Bird

This edition published in 2020 by
Ryland Peters & Small
20–21 Jockey's Fields, London
WC1R 4BW
and 341 E 116th St, New York NY
10029
www.rylandpeters.com

10 9 8 7 6 5 4 3 2 1

First published in 2019

Text copyright © Leah Vanderveldt
2019
Design and photographs copyright
© Ryland Peters & Small 2019

ISBN: 978-1-78879-218-9

Printed in China

A CIP record for this book is
available from the British Library.
US Library of Congress Cataloging-
in-Publication Data has been
applied for.

General recipe notes
• Both British (Metric) and
American (Imperial plus US cups)
measurements are included in these
recipes for your convenience,
however it is important to work
with one set of measurements only
and not alternate between the two
within a recipe.
• All spoon measurements are
level unless otherwise specified.
A teaspoon is 5 ml, a tablespoon
is 15 ml.
• Ovens should be preheated
to the specified temperatures.
We recommend using an oven
thermometer. If using a fan-assisted
oven, adjust temperatures according
to the manufacturer's instructions.
• For infusion recipes, all herbs are
dried unless otherwise indicated.
Aim to buy herbs that are both grown
organically and sourced responsibly.
Mountain Rose Herbs is a great
place to start online but also check
out any local herb shops near you.

Important notes on CBD
• Readers are urged to consult a
relevant and qualified specialist
or physician for individual advice
before taking CBD in conjunction
with any other medical conditions,
medication or if pregnant or
breastfeeding.
• For the purposes of this book,
a single dose of CBD is considered
to be about ¼ teaspoon. However,
it's important to pay attention to
the concentration of the specific oil
you're using, and find what is best
for you. Take note of the amount
that works for you and sub that
in anywhere you see ¼ teaspoon
in the single-serve recipes.
• A non-flavoured oil-based
tincture of CBD is recommended
for use in the recipes in this book.

Disclaimer

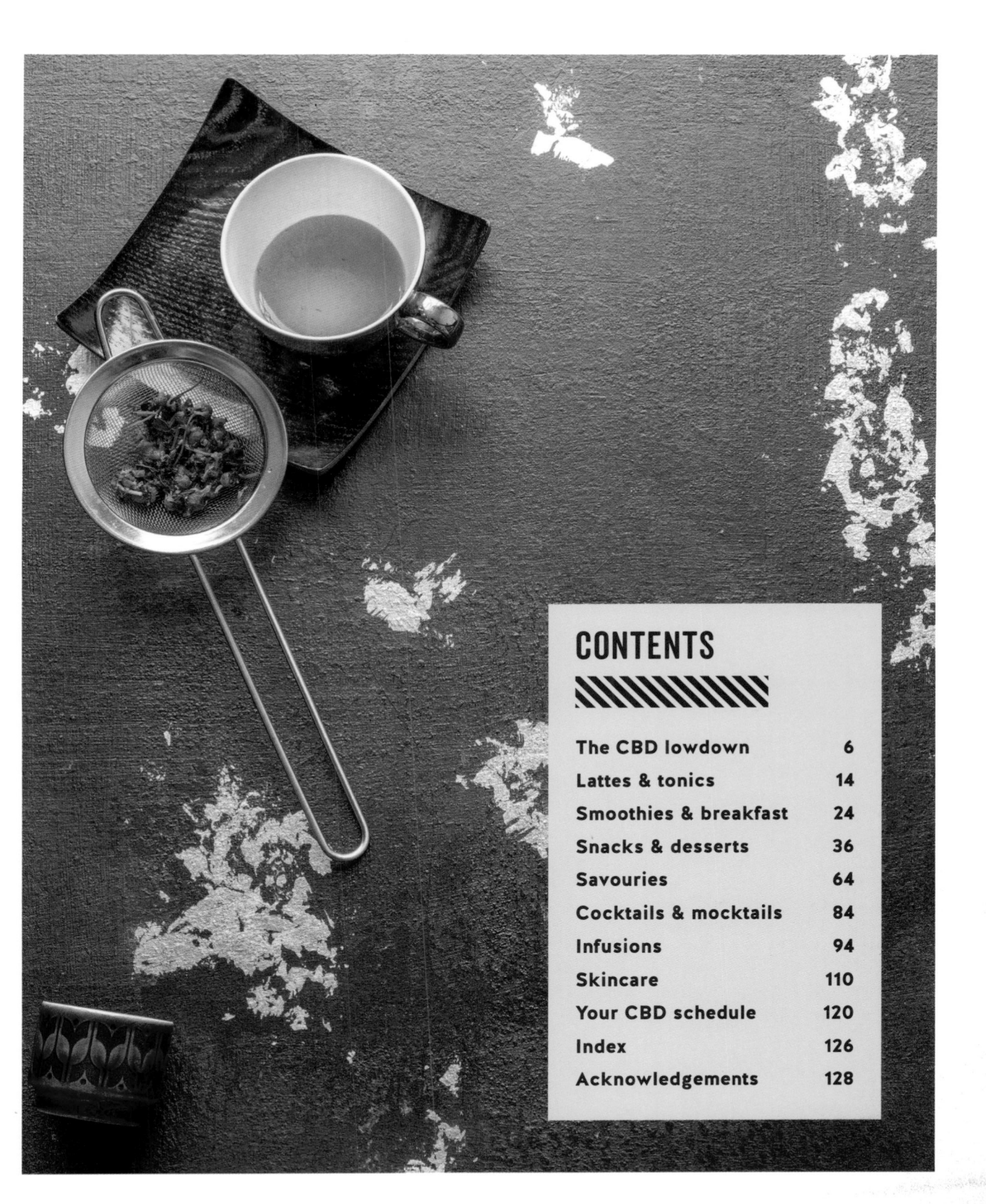

CONTENTS

The CBD lowdown	6
Lattes & tonics	14
Smoothies & breakfast	24
Snacks & desserts	36
Savouries	64
Cocktails & mocktails	84
Infusions	94
Skincare	110
Your CBD schedule	120
Index	126
Acknowledgements	128

THE CBD LOWDOWN

CBD (short for cannabidiol) is a chemical compound found in the hemp plant, a variety of cannabis. As a supplement, it has made waves in the wellness world, primarily due to its potent anti-inflammatory properties. Let's get this question out of the way first: unlike marijuana, CBD does not get you high. Not even a little bit. It does, however, have the potential to alleviate a wide range of medical ailments, from physical pains to mental health. It is purported to have all the benefits of medicinal cannabis, but leave you feeling calm and relaxed rather than stoned. I've seen the benefits firsthand, having taken CBD regularly myself long-term. In this book, I'll lay out the facts and share my insight into CBD, along with some delicious plant-based recipes in which you can try the supplement for yourself.

MY EXPERIENCE

I first heard about CBD oil on a podcast, where they discussed its anti-inflammatory properties and its pain-relief potential. It caught my attention because once a month I was getting some pretty severe, fetal-position-inducing pain on the first day of my period. As someone certified in culinary nutrition, I had tried making more anti-inflammatory food adjustments to my already good diet, but aside from sitting on the couch all day with a heating pad on my stomach and taking too many over-the-counter painkillers, nothing was cutting it. I'm a natural remedy person, and I knew there had to be something else out there for me besides taking pills every few hours, but I had yet to find it.

After a bit of research, I decided on Charlotte's Web Hemp Oil, and gave it a try right away – about a week before my period. That month, the onset of my cramps was significantly less intense (which could be due to several factors), but I decided to take a dose of the oil instead of two Advil and see what happened. It took away my cramps within 30 minutes, the same as a typical over-the-counter pain relief pill. I was hopeful when I first started taking CBD, but still pretty sceptical, so I was genuinely overjoyed when it worked better than I expected. And I started to wonder what else this stuff could do.

ANXIETY

I had also read about some of the other purported benefits of CBD and was interested to see the effects it had – especially on my anxiety levels. I don't have a severe anxiety disorder, but I, like so many people today, often

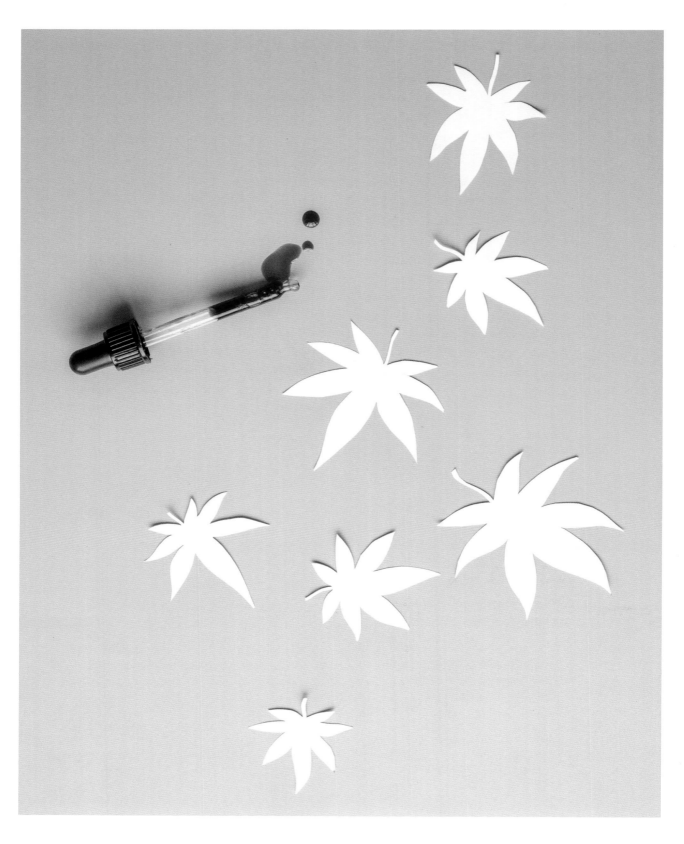

find myself in the grips of anxiety when dealing with everyday stress, unknown social situations or worry. I sometimes lose half a day to an anxiety spiral, trying to alleviate the distracting sensation of a fist of tension in my gut.

The best way I can describe the noticeable difference that CBD has made to my feelings of anxiety is that it diffuses that knotted nervous feeling. That mental spiral I get lost in gradually dissipates until all of a sudden I realize, wow, I feel better. Nothing drastic or intense, just a gentle feeling of well-being. Taking CBD oil has allowed me to shed the feelings that used to consume me or prevent me from going to an event. It gives me a calmer, 'I've got this' kind of feeling that can make a huge difference. I have noticed that regularly taking small amounts has had a cumulative effect on my anxiety overall, and taking a bit more tends to help if I'm having a particularly anxious day.

SLEEP

Linked to my anxiety, my sleep used to be unpredictable, with weeks at a time filled with great sleep and others riddled with random 3am wake-ups or over-active bedtime brain.

So I started taking CBD oil with my tea about an hour before bed and noticed real results. After two years of doing this, I still occasionally get a thought spiral that keeps me up — I am human, after all — but my overall sleep experience has improved drastically.

DEPRESSION

On the other side of that anxiety coin, depression is something I've dealt with throughout my life and it can creep up if I'm not vigilant with my mental health. But since taking CBD oil regularly, depression hasn't been a huge issue for me.

I'm still me, and at times I still get anxious, emotional and blue. CBD isn't a cure-all, but knowing that I have this natural helping hand in my toolbox is comforting.

THE ENDOCANNABINOID SYSTEM & CBD

The endocannabinoid system is a biological system that controls many of the physical responses in our bodies. The system needs to be kept balanced in order for us to maintain a healthy nervous system, brain health, regulate hormones, get good sleep and regulate pain.

The naturally occurring chemicals within the hemp plant contain many cannabinoids or phytocannabinoids, and CBD is one of these. Our endocannabinoid systems have cannabinoid receptors that can make use of extra CBD to help balance our systems. Our bodies are designed to benefit from this chemical compound, and while they produce their own cannabinoids, using CBD oil can help top up and return your endocannabinoid system to equilibrium.

HEALTH BENEFITS IN GENERAL

Though I'm not a doctor or a scientist, my training in culinary nutrition has given me a thorough understanding of wellness supplements and how they interact with our bodies. My view on the potential benefits of CBD comes from having studied the information available, coupled with the fact that having tried it, I have quickly realized what a helpful addition it is in my life.

While the science and studies supporting the use of CBD are promising, they are still in the early stages. A lot of the benefits I mention have been researched, but that research is ongoing. What we do have, though, is strong anecdotal evidence from people who use it and whose lives have been improved by it. Reported benefits include:

- Anti-inflammatory
- Pain management
- Anti-anxiety
- Antidepressant
- Improved sleep
- Antioxidant
- Neuroprotectant
- Brain health
- Heart health
- Arthritis pain

HEMP VS MARIJUANA

As previously mentioned, CBD is a chemical compound found in the hemp plant. Hemp and marijuana are both varieties of the cannabis plant. Those who are new to CBD often mistakenly assume that it will make them feel stoned. It's understandably confusing – CBD comes from the same type of plant as marijuana (the stuff you smoke) and yet, it doesn't give the same drastic sensations.

The main difference between hemp and marijuana is the amount of THC or tetrahydrocannabinol – the chemical component that produces psychoactive effects and gets you high. Hemp only contains trace amounts of THC (less than 0.3 per cent). This important distinction means that hemp is legal to cultivate and sell with a licence in the United States, the UK and many other parts of the world. Marijuana, on the other hand, is mostly illegal around the world, due to its elevated levels of THC. Confusingly, marijuana also contains CBD in varying amounts, but a lot less than the hemp plant.

THC VS CBD

THC and CBD are two of at least 113 phytocannabinoids – the chemical compounds naturally found within the cannabis plant. THC is the psychoactive chemical compound that gets you high or stoned and CBD is the compound that promotes relaxation and reduces bodily stress. Individually and together, they are two of the most powerful compounds. The 'entourage effect' is a term used in the cannabis industry for the positive effects that you get when these two chemical compounds work in harmony together. Therefore, a lot of good-quality CBD oils will contain trace amounts of THC – just enough to enhance the effectiveness of it, but not enough to get you high. These trace amounts of THC are naturally occurring in the plant, and will be present if the oil is a high-quality oil that uses the real plant instead of just extracting the chemicals from it.

CBD OIL VS HEMP SEED OIL

Hemp seed oil and hemp seeds are also available as wellness supplements. Hemp seeds are a good source of omega fatty acids and plant-based protein, but they don't contain phytocannabinoids like CBD. These beneficial compounds of the plant are found largely in the flowers of the plant, not the seeds. CBD oil is made from the whole plant (leaves, stem and flowers), as opposed to the seeds.

When you're taking a hemp oil like CBD that contains the flowers of the plant, you're getting those potent extra benefits that promote calm and quell inflammation.

WAYS TO TAKE IT

CBD is available in a few different forms – capsules, topical creams and sprays, smokable oils for vapes and oil-based tinctures. I prefer the oil to capsules. With the oil-based tincture, you can take it under the tongue or put it in food and drink, as we'll explore here.

THE OIL BASE

The oil-based tincture is one of the most popular ways of taking CBD, because the CBD is more easily absorbed into the body when delivered along with fat. Many tinctures will blend the CBD with either MCT oil or olive oil. For the purposes of this book, I use a non-flavoured oil-based tincture. The oil-based tincture usually comes in a dark-coloured stopper bottle.

WHERE DO I BUY IT?

CBD oil for medicinal use is legal in all 50 United States and the UK, and it is becoming legal in other countries as well. I typically buy mine online because, well, I buy pretty much everything online these days. But you can find it in specialized health stores and through some alternative health practitioners like acupuncturists. Because CBD is becoming such big business but is still largely unregulated, there are a lot of sketchy products on the market. To make sure you're getting a good-quality product that you'll be able to reap the benefits of, below are my top tips.

WHAT TO LOOK FOR WHEN BUYING CBD

- Note the concentration of CBD and the recommended dosage. A lot of brands sell different levels of potency in their range of tinctures, and all tinctures vary in their concentration level. Buy the lowest potency available to start with and build up from there. If a bottle doesn't have the amount of

CBD listed on its label, chances are it's low quality and contains very small amounts.

- Go for 'full spectrum' or 'whole food' CBD hemp oil. These terms mean that all the different parts of the plant have been used (leaves, flowers and stem). These contain beneficial terpenes, flavonoids and a variety of phytocannabinoids, in addition to CBD.
- Look for 'organically grown' and 'non-GMO'. There's no widespread regulation for this yet, so it's difficult to get an official certification, but take note of the omission of growing practices when looking for an oil and go with a brand that's explicit about how their product is grown.
- Opt for products that are open about where their plants are grown, and make sure that growing hemp is legal in that place. There are a lot of good brands coming out of Colorado and California, where both hemp and marijuana are legalized and regulated. If they can't tell you where the farms are, you probably don't want it.
- Look for 'third party tested'. Any brand that will happily provide consumers with lab results of the chemical breakdown of their product is the way to go. Transparency is key in this unregulated market.

Brands I recommend include: Charlotte's Web, RITUAL, CW Hemp, Humboldt Apothecary, Lily CBD, Soul Addict, Mineral Health Robyn and Rosebud. But this isn't an exhaustive list and there are new brands popping up all the time. Do your own research and find a product that you trust.

HOW MUCH TO TAKE

As mentioned in my list of tips on what to look for when buying CBD (left), you should note the concentration of the type of oil you're buying and start small with your dose. You can then work your way up gradually and see how you feel. I would consider a low dose to be around 10–15 mg per day and a high dose about 40 mg and above per day. I take somewhere between 20–30 mg (¼–½ teaspoon) per day of the particular potency I use, sometimes more when I find myself really anxious about something or am having intense cramps. Any less than 20 mg and I can't really notice the effects, but you might find that something different works better for you depending on what you're treating and the way your body works. Check in with yourself regularly when you take it and take note of your sweet spot. I would advise taking a maximum of up to 50–60 mg per day, you can't exactly overdose on it but, like anything, too much might make you feel unwell (and do read the note on page 4 before taking CBD oil).

I use CBD oil most days and believe that the anti-inflammatory benefits are cumulative. But some days I don't take it, or I'll go a period of time without it and that's fine too. Like everything health-related, my philosophy is do what feels right for you.

WHY COOK WITH IT?

The main reason people add CBD oil to food and drink is to make it more palatable – the herbal flavour can be quite strong, so many people have a tough time taking it straight up. You can hide the herbal taste or play to it by adding lots of complementary flavours. Cooking with CBD is also useful for spacing out small measures throughout the day, and it provides an enjoyable way to take your dose.

HOW TO COOK WITH IT

In this book, we'll be using CBD oil without any flavours added (some brands sell oils flavoured with things like mint chocolate). As a general rule, don't heat the oil above 180°C/350°F, as the potency will degrade.

I consider a single dose to be about ¼ teaspoon and the recipes in this book reflect this. However, it's important to pay attention to the concentration of the specific oil you're using, find what works best for you and sub that in anywhere you see ¼ teaspoon in the single-serve recipes if needed. Larger batches may take a little calculating, but hopefully won't be too difficult.

A HOLISTIC EXPERIENCE

CBD isn't a miracle worker, although it might sound like it sometimes. It's simply one tool that you can have in reserve for keeping your body and mind healthy. If you suffer from chronic pain, look at other changes you can make to your everyday diet and try to incorporate other ingredients with anti-inflammatory properties. If your diet is rich in dark leafy vegetables, legumes, fruit and nuts, you are on the right track. Adding extra anti-inflammatory ingredients like black pepper, cayenne pepper, turmeric and ginger whenever you can is also highly beneficial. Keeping consumption of refined carbohydrates, sugar, trans fats and too much alcohol to a minimum can also be helpful.

If you're taking CBD to help with the ups and downs of riding that anxiety roller coaster, I strongly suggest adopting CBD alongside a varied routine that includes other holistic anti-anxiety practices, such as mindfulness/ meditation, journaling, exercise and spending time outside.

You won't change your entire life just by taking CBD, but once you start seeing some results from taking it, it may well give you the motivation you need to make other small changes that will make you feel better overall.

I see CBD oil as a useful supplement that can help get me back to neutral. I use it to enhance the state of well-being that I'm working towards each day.

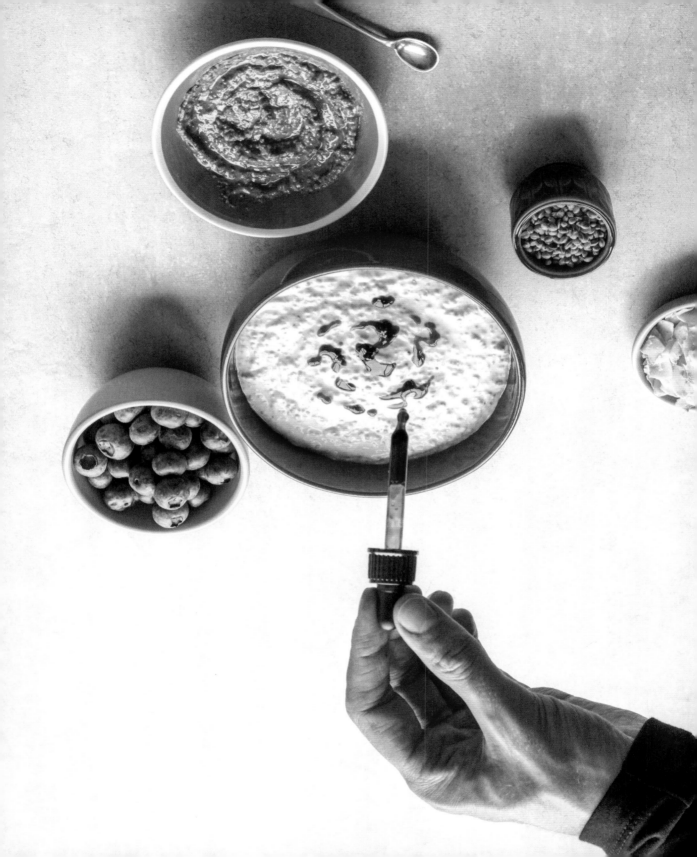

LATTES & TONICS

Revitalizing and relaxing CBD beverages to enjoy morning, afternoon or evening.

CBD TURMERIC LATTE

//////////////////

This one is for night-time relaxing – I've actually heard versions of this recipe called Moon Milk. Were you ever given warm milk to help you sleep as a kid? This is a version of that comforting drink with an anti-inflammatory boost.

235 ml/1 cup plant-based milk
   (I like almond or coconut)
1 teaspoon coconut butter
½ teaspoon ground turmeric
¼ teaspoon ground cardamom
¼ teaspoon ground cinnamon
pinch of freshly ground black
   pepper
1–1½ teaspoons agave syrup
¼ teaspoon CBD oil

SERVES 1

Place the milk in a small saucepan set over a low heat. Once the milk has warmed through and is starting to bubble at the edges, add the coconut butter, turmeric, cardamom, cinnamon, black pepper and agave syrup and whisk together. Increase the heat a little and simmer, whisking regularly, for about 5 minutes. Remove from the heat and whisk in the CBD oil. Pour into a mug and enjoy hot.

CBD ROSE
LATTE

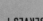

This rose latte is another soothing drink, good for any time of the day. Using rooibos tea in this recipe makes it naturally caffeine-free and the slightly sweet floral flavour of rosewater adds something special. I order food-grade rose petals online, but you can find them in gourmet or speciality shops too.

175 ml/¾ cup boiled water
1 vanilla rooibos tea bag
60 ml/¼ cup plant-based milk
of your choice
½ teaspoon rosewater
agave syrup, to taste
¼ teaspoon CBD oil
food-grade dried rose petals,
to serve (optional)

SERVES 1

Start by pouring the boiled water over the vanilla rooibos tea bag in a mug. Leave it to brew for 10 minutes.

Meanwhile, combine the milk and rosewater in a small saucepan over a low-medium heat and let warm through for about 5 minutes until just hot. Remove and discard the rooibos tea bag and add the brewed tea to the saucepan of milk. Stir in agave syrup, to taste, followed by the CBD oil. Pour the rose latte into a mug and top with a few dried rose petals to serve, if you like.

CBD MATCHA LATTE

I love matcha for the low-key energy boost it provides. The caffeine in this powdered form of green tea gives a calmer form of energy release, making it great for pairing with CBD oil. Serving this drink cold over ice is my preference, but it's nice served warm, too.

175 ml/¾ cup coconut milk
60 ml/¼ cup filtered water
1–2 teaspoons matcha powder
¼ teaspoon CBD oil
1–2 teaspoons maple syrup
  (optional)
ice, to serve (optional)

SERVES 1

Combine the ingredients in a blender and process until well combined.

Serve the latte over ice in a tall glass, or warm through on the hob/stovetop and serve in a mug.

CBD BEETROOT LATTE

While beetroot/beet powder is available, I always like to use the real thing when I can. Beetroot/beet is a powerful liver-protectant that contains potent anti-inflammatory and antioxidant properties; it gives an earthy flavour to this sweet, spiced latte.

235 ml/1 cup coconut milk
1 small ready-prepared steamed
  and peeled beetroot/beet
60 ml/¼ cup filtered water
1 teaspoon coconut sugar
½ teaspoon ground cinnamon
¼ teaspoon ground ginger
¼ teaspoon vanilla extract
¼ teaspoon CBD oil

SERVES 1

Place half the coconut milk in a small saucepan over a low-medium heat and bring gently to the point of almost boiling.

Meanwhile, combine the beetroot/beet, remaining half of the coconut milk, the water, coconut sugar, cinnamon, ginger, vanilla and CBD oil in a blender and process on high for 1–2 minutes until completely smooth and frothy. Pour the beetroot/beet mixture into your serving cup. Note: If your blender isn't powerful enough to completely liquefy your beet mixture, pass it through a fine-mesh sieve/strainer before adding to your serving cup.

Rinse out the blender and add the hot coconut milk. Process again to froth the coconut milk a little. Pour the frothed milk into the beet mixture and serve immediately.

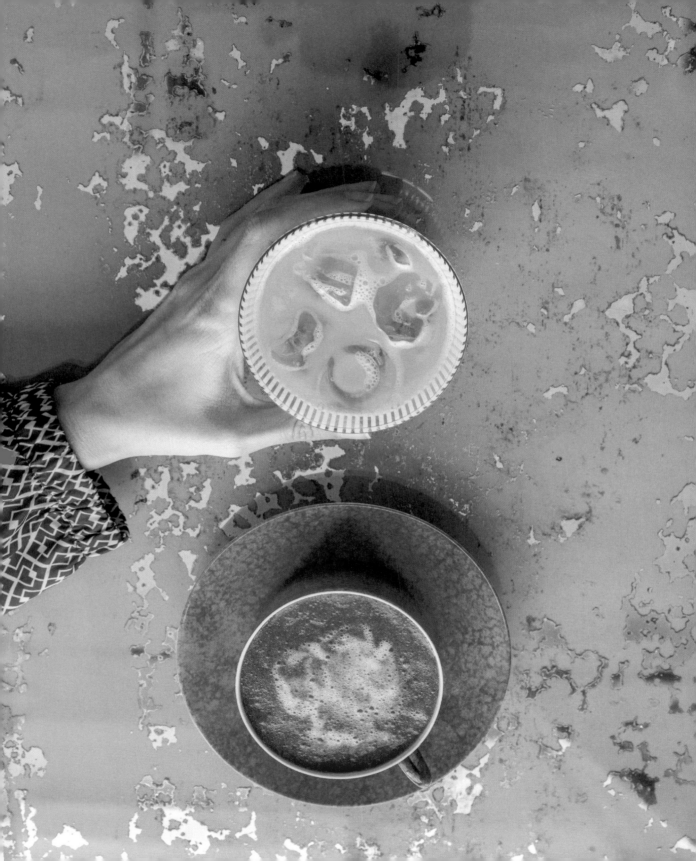

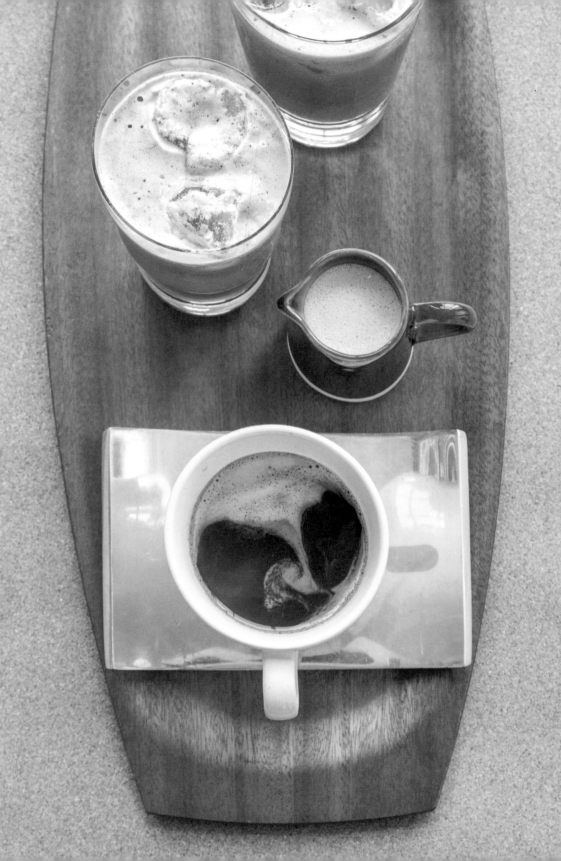

CBD DANDELION ICED COFFEE TONIC

//////////////

Caffeine-free roasted dandelion root is an excellent coffee replacement – the roasting process gives it a coffee-like quality. Whether you're looking to cut back on caffeine or just find yourself in the mood for an iced coffee at 4pm but don't want to mess with your sleep cycle, dandelion root is a great alternative that also promotes liver health. I have added lion's mane mushroom powder to this blend for an extra brain boost and to help keep you going throughout your day.

235 ml/1 cup cooled strong-brewed
    roasted dandelion tea or
    2 teaspoons roasted dandelion
    root powder mixed with 235 ml/
    1 cup cold water
1 tablespoon coconut butter,
    melted
1 teaspoon lion's mane mushroom
    powder (optional)
1 teaspoon hemp seeds
¼ teaspoon CBD oil
maple syrup, to taste
ice, to serve

SERVES 1

Combine all the ingredients in a blender and process at high speed until completely liquid.

    Pour over ice into a glass and serve.

CBD COFFEE TONIC

//////////////

The added fibre and fat in this coffee ward off any possible negative effects of caffeine on an empty stomach, and let you enjoy a rich, sweet morning beverage. Chaga mushrooms (an optional extra) are antioxidant powerhouses.

2 tablespoons raw cashews
1 tablespoon coconut butter,
    melted
1 large Medjool date, pitted
¼ teaspoon CBD oil
1 teaspoon chaga mushroom
    powder (optional)
175–235 ml/¾–1 cup hot water
175 ml/¾ cup hot freshly brewed
    coffee

SERVES 1

Combine all the ingredients (apart from the coffee) in a blender and process until completely smooth. If you don't have a high-speed blender you may need to strain the liquid. Pour the freshly brewed coffee into a mug and top with the cashew milk. Enjoy hot.

    Tip: If you don't have a high-speed blender, soak the cashews and date for at least an hour or overnight to soften before blending.

CBD HOT CACAO

////////////

This is one of my favourite afternoon pick-me-ups. It is simple to prepare and makes me feel like I'm really treating myself.

235 ml/1 cup plant-based milk of your choice
2 tablespoons raw cacao powder
1–1½ teaspoons maple syrup
¼ teaspoon CBD oil
pinch of sea salt

SERVES 1

Place the milk in a small saucepan over a low heat. Once the milk has warmed through and is starting to bubble at the edges, whisk in the cacao powder. Increase the heat a little and simmer, stirring often, for 3–4 minutes.

Remove the pan from the heat and whisk in the maple syrup, CBD oil and sea salt. Pour the hot cacao into a mug and enjoy.

CBD CHAI LATTE

////////////

If I wasn't so completely in love with my morning coffee, I would be a morning chai person. I love the combination of the warming spices with milk, which makes for an extra-special creamy treat. If you want to make it caffeine-free, swap the black tea for rooibos.

1 teaspoon ground cinnamon
1 teaspoon ground ginger
½ teaspoon ground cardamom
½ teaspoon ground cloves
pinch of freshly ground black pepper
1 tablespoon black loose-leaf tea
agave syrup, to taste
¼ teaspoon CBD oil per serving
120 ml/½ cup unsweetened plant-based milk of your choice

SERVES 2

To make the chai spice blend, combine the cinnamon, ginger, cardamom, cloves and black pepper in a small bowl or jar and mix well to combine.

In a small saucepan, combine 1 tablespoon of the spice blend with the black tea and 500 ml/2 cups of water. Bring to the boil, then reduce the heat and simmer gently for 10 minutes.

Sieve/strain the chai tea through a tea strainer or fine-mesh sieve/strainer into two mugs. Stir in agave syrup, to taste, followed by the CBD oil.

Rinse out the small saucepan and add the milk. Heat through for 3 minutes until warm. Divide the warm milk between the mugs and serve immediately.

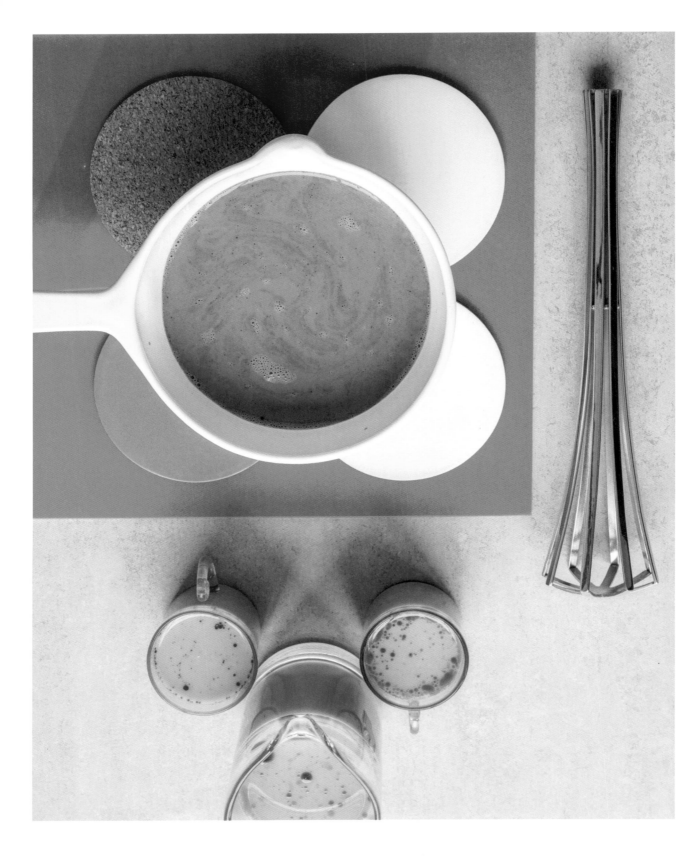

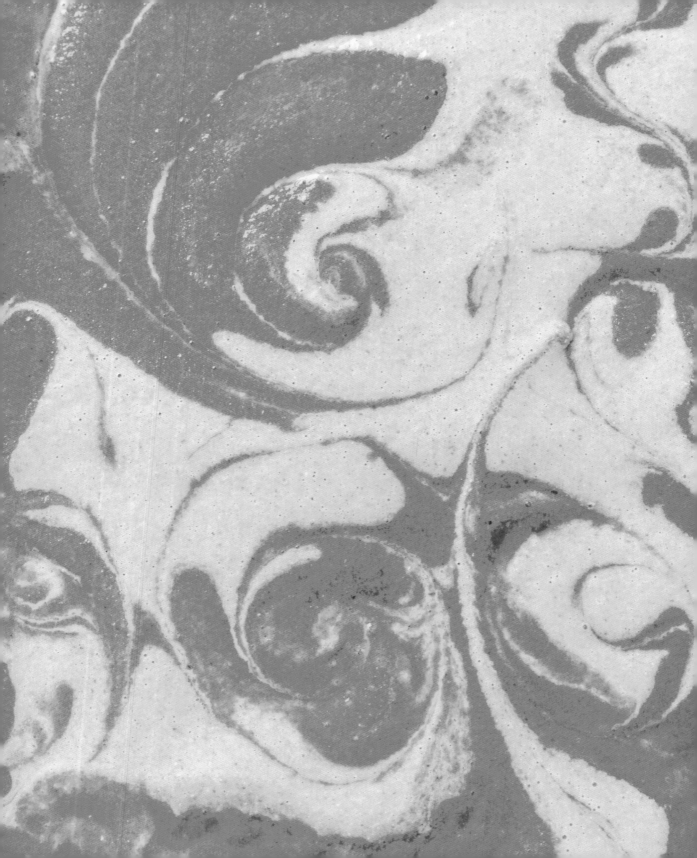

SMOOTHIES & BREAKFAST

Start your day in a delicious way, and with an anti-inflammatory boost.

CBD GREEN STRAWBERRY SMOOTHIE

////////////

This smoothie is perfect for keeping your energy levels up all morning – it contains fruit, a vegetable and some healthy fat and protein from the almond butter and pumpkin seeds/ pepitas. I love these little seeds – just a tablespoon a day can help keep your hormones in check.

355 ml/1½ cups plant-based milk of your choice
190 g/1 cup frozen strawberries
½ frozen banana, peeled
150 g/1 scant cup frozen spinach
1 tablespoon pumpkin seeds/ pepitas
1–2 tablespoons natural (no added sugar) peanut or almond butter
¼ teaspoon CBD oil

SERVES 1

Combine all the ingredients in a blender and process until smooth.

CBD BEET BERRY SMOOTHIE

////////////

Beets are an incredibly iron-rich vegetable and they help to keep our hearts healthy. For these reasons, they also help us to perform and recover more efficiently from intense exercise. Paired with the anti-inflammatory properties of CBD, the two make a perfect replenishing post-exercise drink.

235 ml/1 cup coconut milk
60 ml/¼ cup filtered water
2 small ready-prepared steamed and peeled beetroots/beets
125 g/½ cup frozen raspberries
95 g/½ cup frozen strawberries
95 g/½ cup frozen cauliflower florets
1 tablespoon natural (no added sugar) almond butter
¼ teaspoon vanilla extract or vanilla pod/bean powder
¼ teaspoon CBD oil

SERVES 1

Combine all the ingredients in a blender and process until smooth.

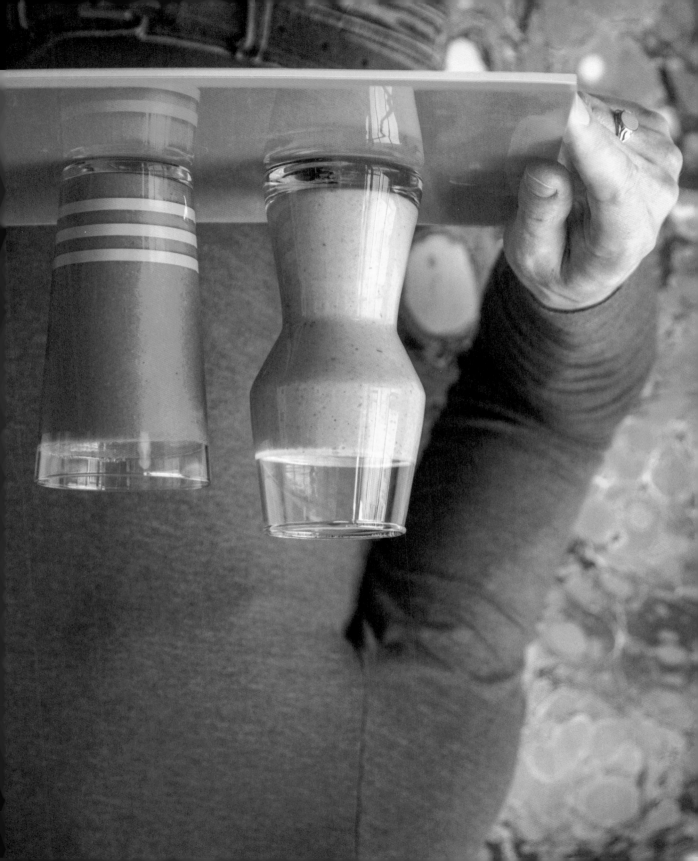

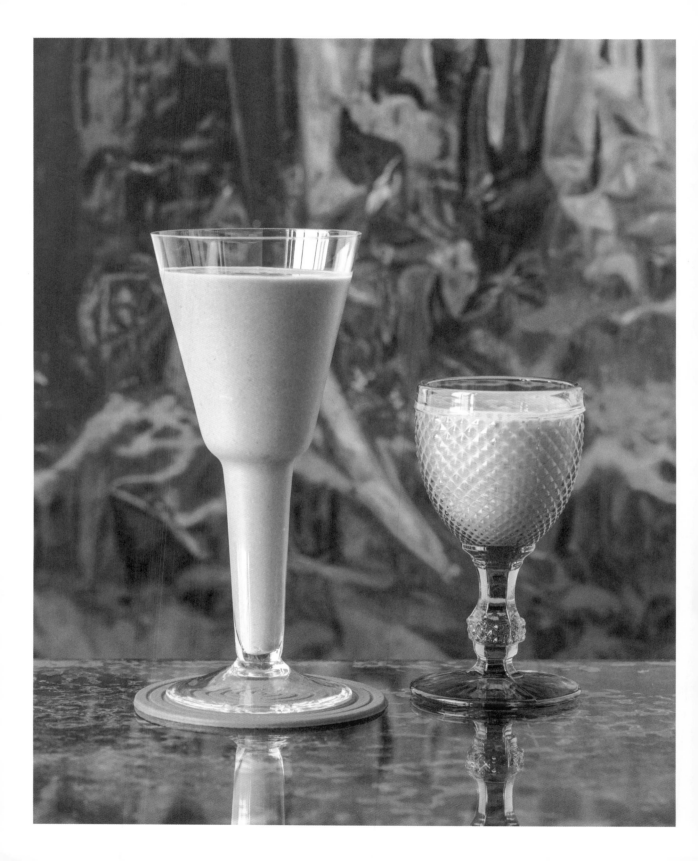

CBD CHOCOLATE & PEANUT BUTTER SMOOTHIE

////////////

This is a healthier spin on a chocolate and peanut butter milkshake. I love combining cacao with CBD oil (as you'll see throughout this book!) because both work so well for calming the body – with cacao's magnesium levels and CBD's anti-inflammatory qualities.

355 ml/1½ cups coconut
   or almond milk
1½ frozen bananas, peeled
115 g/4 oz. frozen cauliflower
   florets
2 tablespoons cacao powder
1–2 tablespoons peanut butter
¼ teaspoon CBD oil

SERVES 1

Combine all the ingredients in a blender and process until smooth. Enjoy.

CBD BANANA & CINNAMON SMOOTHIE

////////////

I couldn't help adding a sneaky vegetable into this simple and classic smoothie combination. With the sweetness of banana and cinnamon, a little frozen cauliflower goes by undetected and adds to the nutrient content and creamy texture.

1½ frozen bananas, peeled
95 g/½ cup frozen cauliflower
   florets
355 ml/1½ cups plant-based milk
   of your choice
1 tablespoon chia seeds
½ teaspoon ground cinnamon
¼ teaspoon CBD oil
pinch of ground nutmeg, to serve

SERVES 1

Combine all the ingredients (apart from the nutmeg) in a blender and process until smooth. Top with the pinch of nutmeg and serve.

CBD MANGO & GINGER SMOOTHIE

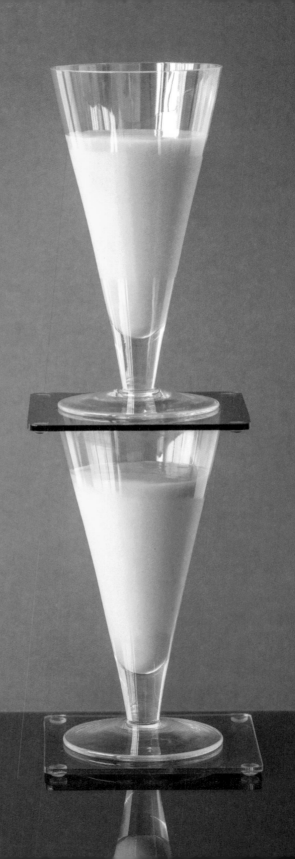

I love this bright smoothie for when my stomach needs soothing or I feel a cold coming on. It's packed with healthy fats, fibre and cure-all ginger to keep you feeling good.

225 g/8 oz. frozen mango
2.5-cm/1-inch piece of fresh
    ginger, peeled
½ avocado, pitted and peeled
freshly squeezed juice of ½ lemon
235 ml/1 cup filtered water
60 ml/¼ cup coconut milk
¼ teaspoon CBD oil

SERVES 1

Combine all the ingredients in a blender and process until smooth. Add more liquid if you prefer a thinner consistency. Serve.

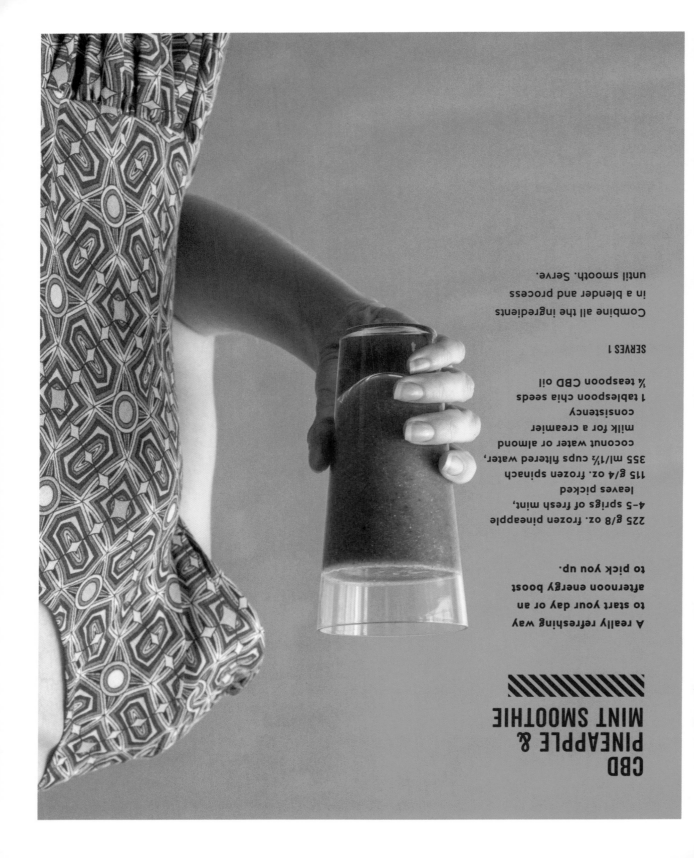

CBD PINEAPPLE & MINT SMOOTHIE

A really refreshing way to start your day or an afternoon energy boost to pick you up.

225 g/8 oz. frozen pineapple
4–5 sprigs of fresh mint, leaves picked
115 g/4 oz. frozen spinach
355 ml/1½ cups filtered water, coconut water or almond milk for a creamier consistency
1 tablespoon chia seeds
¾ teaspoon CBD oil

SERVES 1

Combine all the ingredients in a blender and process until smooth. Serve.

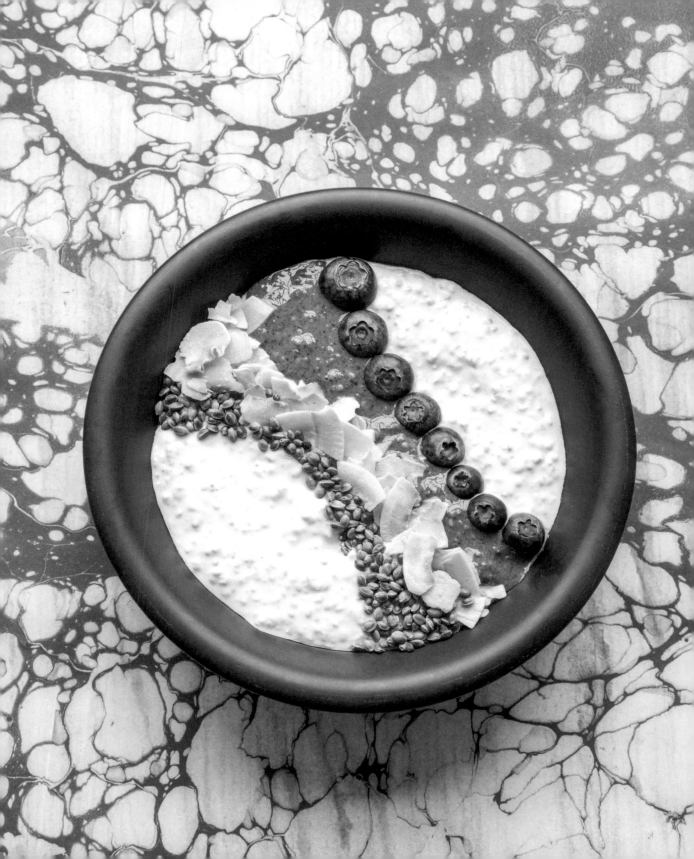

CBD SUPER-POWERED YOGURT BOWL

///////////////

I like to make this recipe the night before so that breakfast is waiting for me in the morning. You can even make three or four of these yogurt bowls for the week ahead and place them in individual jars in the refrigerator. Don't add the CBD oil until the last minute though.

25 g/¼ cup rolled/old-fashioned
   oats
2 tablespoons chia seeds
215 g/1 cup plain plant-based
   yogurt
1 teaspoon maple syrup, to taste
splash of almond or coconut milk
   (optional)
¼ teaspoon CBD oil

OPTIONAL TOPPINGS
natural (no added sugar)
   almond butter
berries or other fresh fruit
toasted coconut flakes
hemp seeds
granola

SERVES 1

Combine the oats, chia seeds, yogurt and maple syrup in a medium bowl. Stir to mix everything together. You can add a splash of milk if you don't want your mixture to be super thick.

Place the mixture in a jar or simply cover the bowl and refrigerate for a minimum of 1 hour or overnight.

When you're ready to serve, stir in the CBD oil, then top with an array of your favourite toppings.

CBD SNACKING GRANOLA CLUSTERS

///////////

A great breakfast snack to take on the road with you. The key to getting good clusters here is having a strict no-stir policy once the granola mixture is on the baking sheet, both during and after baking, until it is totally cold.

95 g/1 cup rolled/old-fashioned oats
25 g/½ cup dried coconut flakes
70 g/½ cup walnuts
35 g/¼ cup pumpkin seeds/pepitas
2 tablespoons chia seeds
2 tablespoons coconut sugar
1 teaspoon ground cinnamon
¼ teaspoon salt
60 ml/¼ cup olive oil
60 ml/¼ cup maple syrup
2 teaspoons CBD oil

baking sheet, lined with baking parchment

MAKES 6 SERVINGS

Preheat the oven to 160°C (325°F) Gas 3.

Combine the oats, coconut flakes, walnuts, pumpkin seeds/pepitas, chia seeds, coconut sugar, cinnamon and salt in a large bowl. Stir to combine and coat everything in cinnamon sugar.

In a separate small bowl, stir together the olive oil, maple syrup and CBD oil. Pour the CBD mixture into the oat mixture, stirring with a rubber spatula until all the ingredients are evenly combined.

Spread the mixture out on the lined baking sheet in an even layer and bake in the preheated oven for 20 minutes. Rotate the baking sheet, then bake for another 15–20 minutes until the granola is just golden. (Again, don't be tempted to stir at any point during baking or after it comes out of the oven.)

Remove the baking sheet from the oven and let the granola cool completely before breaking apart into clusters. These will keep in an airtight container for up to 1 month refrigerated.

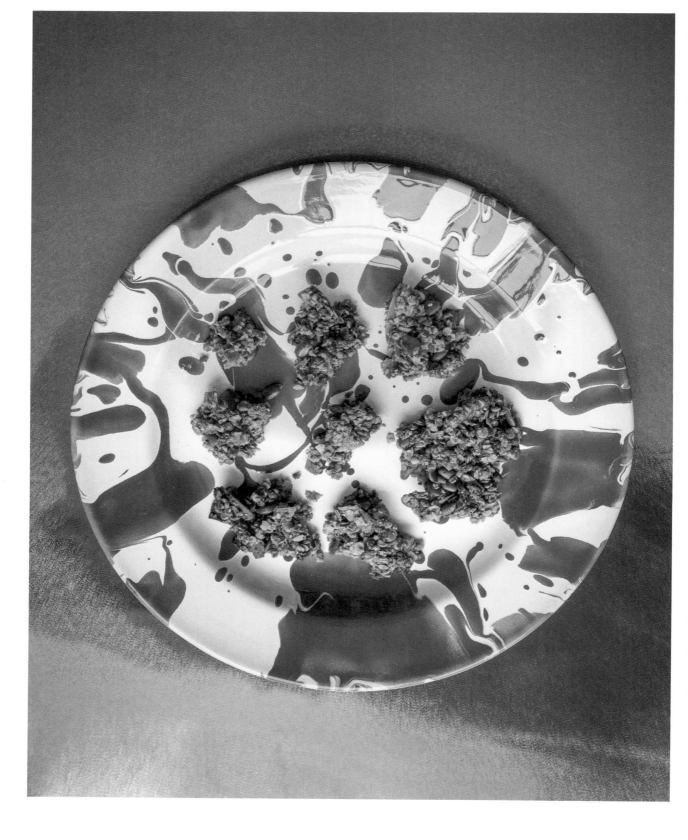

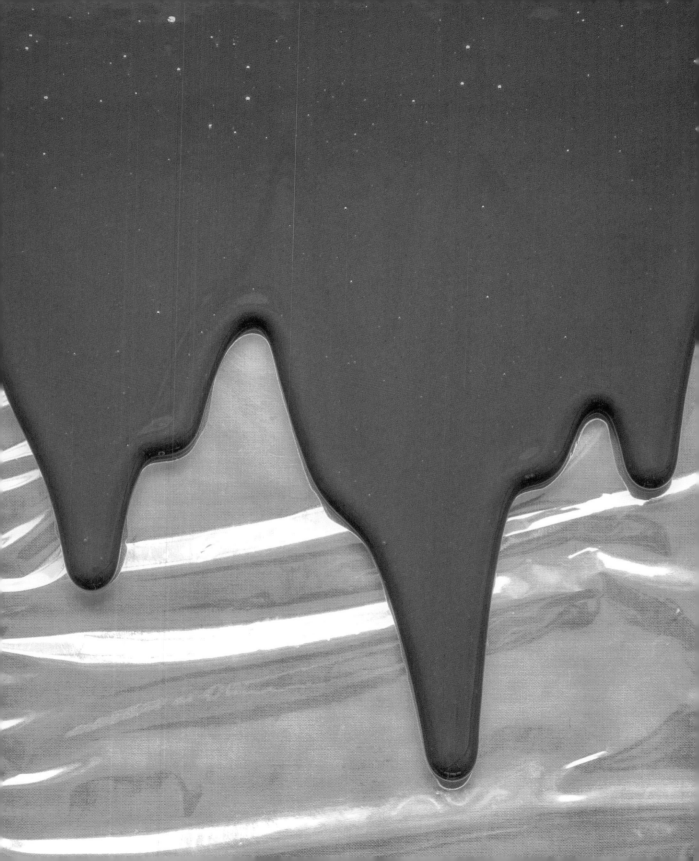

SNACKS & DESSERTS

Sweet and relaxing small
treats to enjoy at home
or on the go.

CBD RAW BROWNIE BITES

As you can see from this chapter, I'm a little obsessed with 'bites'. Basically a healthier take on a chocolate truffle, bites are small sweet treats made from whole foods. They're great for packing loads of superfoods and plant-based medicines like CBD oil into convenient and tasty bite-sized snacks.

10 Medjool dates, pitted
25 g/½ cup dried coconut flakes
2 teaspoons CBD oil
1 teaspoon vanilla extract
50 g/½ cup cacao powder
sea salt, to taste

large plate lined with baking parchment

MAKES 12 BITES/1–2 BITES PER SERVING

Place all the ingredients in a food processor or blender in the order listed and process on a low speed until all the ingredients are well combined and start coming together into a dough of sorts. You may have to scrape down the sides of your machine with a rubber spatula once or twice to achieve a well-mixed situation.

Scoop out the mixture and roll into ping-pong sized balls. Sprinkle with extra sea salt flakes, if desired. Place the bites on the lined plate and put into the freezer for 20 minutes to firm up.

Transfer the brownie bites to a sealable container and refrigerate until needed. They will keep for up to 1 month.

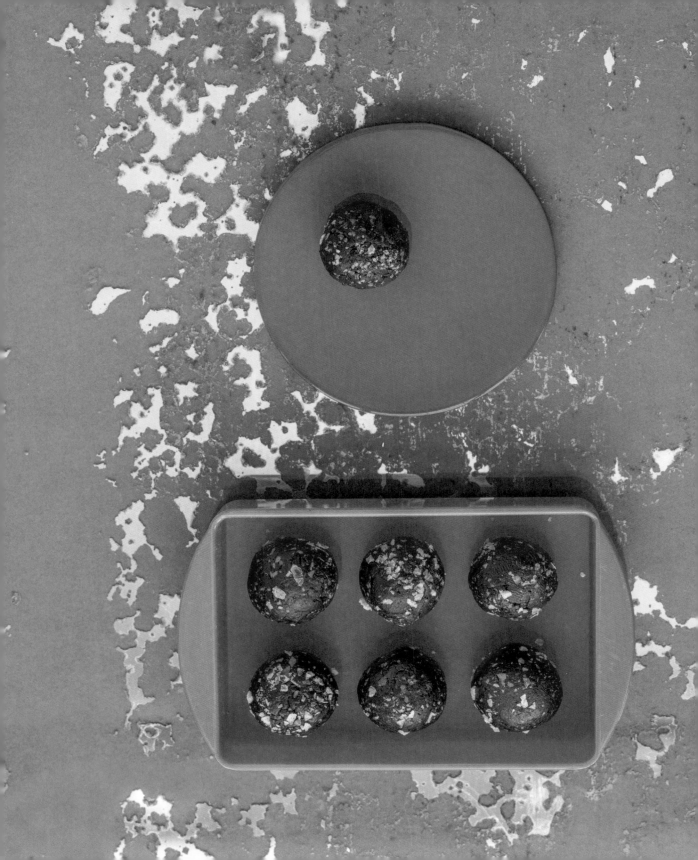

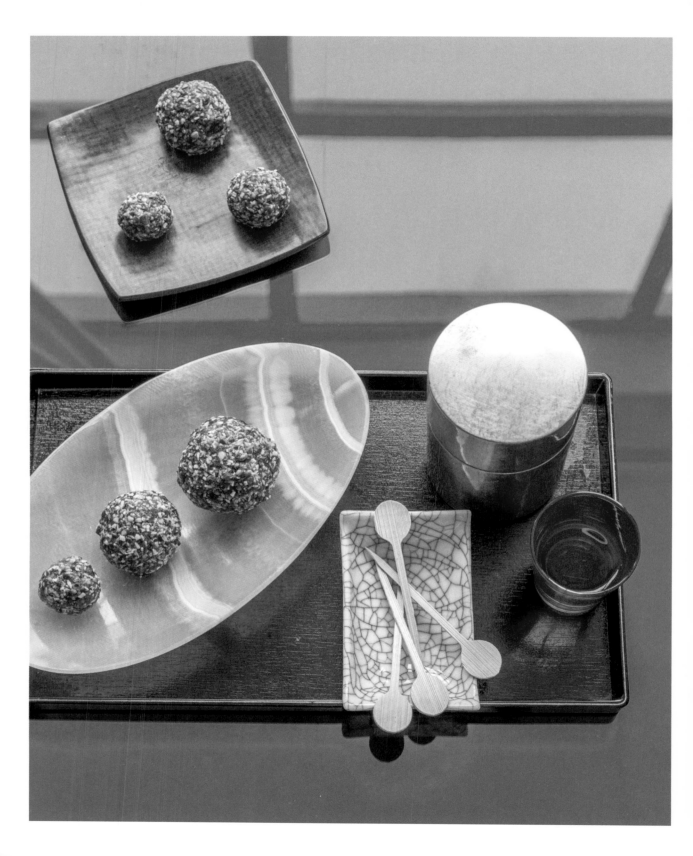

CBD COCONUT & PECAN BITES

Pecan pie meet energy bites – I love to have these little snacks on stand by, especially as the weather gets colder when their autumnal flavours make a welcome treat.

10 Medjool dates, pitted
115 g/1 cup raw pecans
75 g/1 cup desiccated/dried
   shredded coconut
1 teaspoon ground cinnamon
2 tablespoons hemp seeds
1 teaspoon CBD oil
¼ teaspoon sea salt

large plate lined with baking parchment

MAKES 10–12/2 BITES PER SERVING

Combine all the ingredients in a food processor or blender and process until everything is finely chopped and well combined into a dough of sorts, scraping down the sides of the machine one or twice as you go.

Scoop out the mixture and roll into ping-pong sized balls. Place the bites on the lined plate and put into the freezer for 20 minutes to firm up.

Transfer the bites to a sealable container and refrigerate until needed. They will keep for up to 1 month.

CBD PISTACHIO & TAHINI BITES

////////////

Tahini is one of my favourite ingredients. Made from ground sesame seeds, it's a grown-up alternative to peanut butter and is great in both savoury and sweet dishes. When combined with dates, cacao and pistachios, these little bites have tons of unexpected and addictive flavour.

8 Medjool dates, pitted
110 g/½ cup tahini
25 g/⅓ cup desiccated/dried shredded coconut, plus extra for decorating (optional)
45 g/⅓ cup shelled unsalted pistachios
25 g/¼ cup cacao powder
1 teaspoon CBD oil
⅛ teaspoon sea salt

large plate lined with baking parchment

MAKES 9–10/2 BITES PER SERVING

Combine all the ingredients (apart from the extra coconut) in a food processor or high-speed blender and process until you have a well combined dough of sorts, scraping down the sides of the machine one or twice as you go.

Scoop out the mixture and roll into ping-pong sized balls. Roll each ball in a little extra coconut to decorate, if desired. Place the bites on the lined plate and put into the freezer for 20 minutes to firm up.

Transfer the bites to a sealable container and refrigerate until needed. They will keep for up to 1 month.

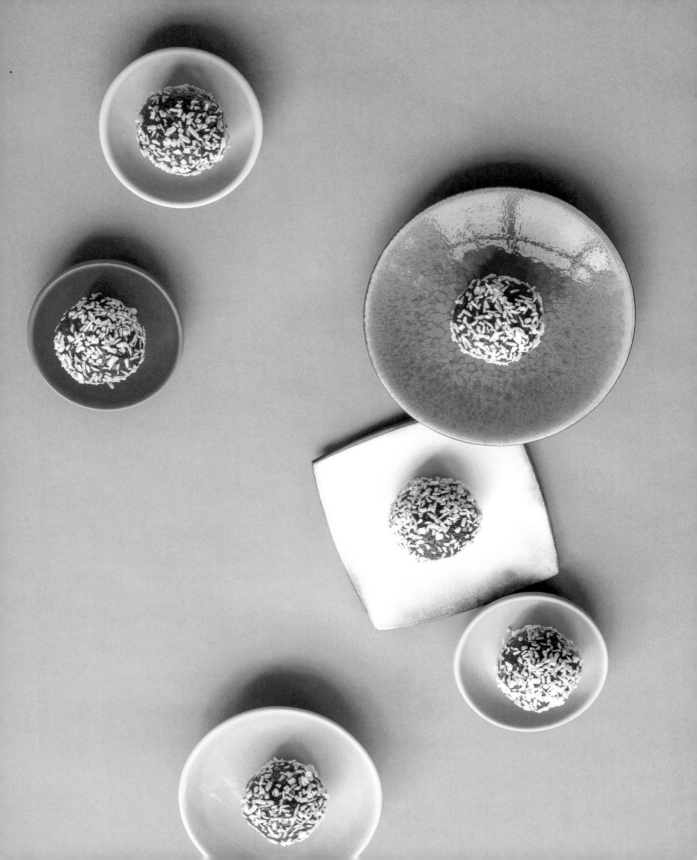

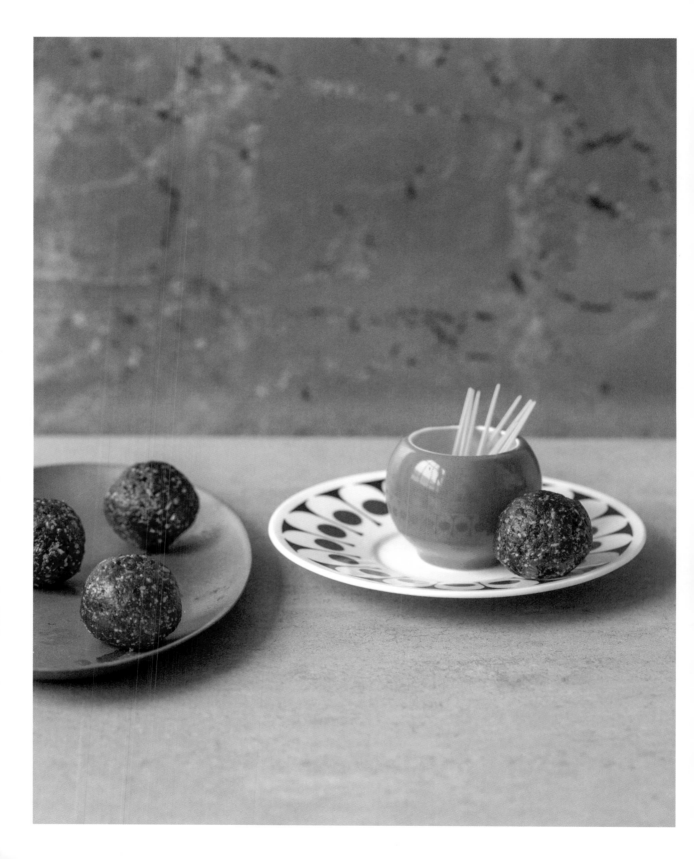

CBD MINT CHOCOLATE BITES

//////////////

These taste a bit like the store-bought Thin Mint cookies you might have had as a kid, but the ingredients they contain are so much better for you.

10 Medjool dates, pitted
110 g/½ cup natural (no added sugar) almond butter
25 g/⅓ cup desiccated/dried shredded coconut
½ teaspoon peppermint extract
3 tablespoons cacao powder or cocoa powder
1 teaspoon CBD oil

large plate lined with baking parchment

MAKES 9–10/2 BITES PER SERVING

Combine all the ingredients in a food processor or blender and process until everything is finely chopped and well combined into a dough of sorts, scraping down the sides of the machine one or twice as you go.

Scoop out the mixture and roll into ping-pong sized balls. Place the bites on the lined plate and put into the freezer for 20 minutes to firm up.

Transfer the bites to a sealable container and refrigerate until needed. They will keep for up to 1 month.

CBD RAW OATMEAL COOKIE BITES

////////////

A cross between cookie dough and a chewy oatmeal cookie, these bites also pack a good protein boost from the almond butter.

50 g/½ cup rolled/old-fashioned oats
75 g/⅓ cup natural (no added sugar) almond butter
2 teaspoons maple syrup
1 teaspoon ground cinnamon
½ teaspoon vanilla extract
sea salt
1½ teaspoons CBD oil
1 teaspoon coconut oil, melted
55 g/2 oz. vegan dark/bittersweet chocolate, chopped or raisins

large plate lined with baking parchment

MAKES 6/1 BITE PER SERVING

Place all the ingredients in a food processor or blender in the order listed and process on a low speed until all the ingredients are well combined and start coming together into a dough of sorts, scraping down the sides of the machine once or twice as you go.

Scoop out the mixture and roll into ping-pong sized balls. Place the bites on the lined plate and put into the freezer for 20 minutes to firm up.

Transfer the bites to a sealable container and refrigerate until needed. They will keep for up to 1 month.

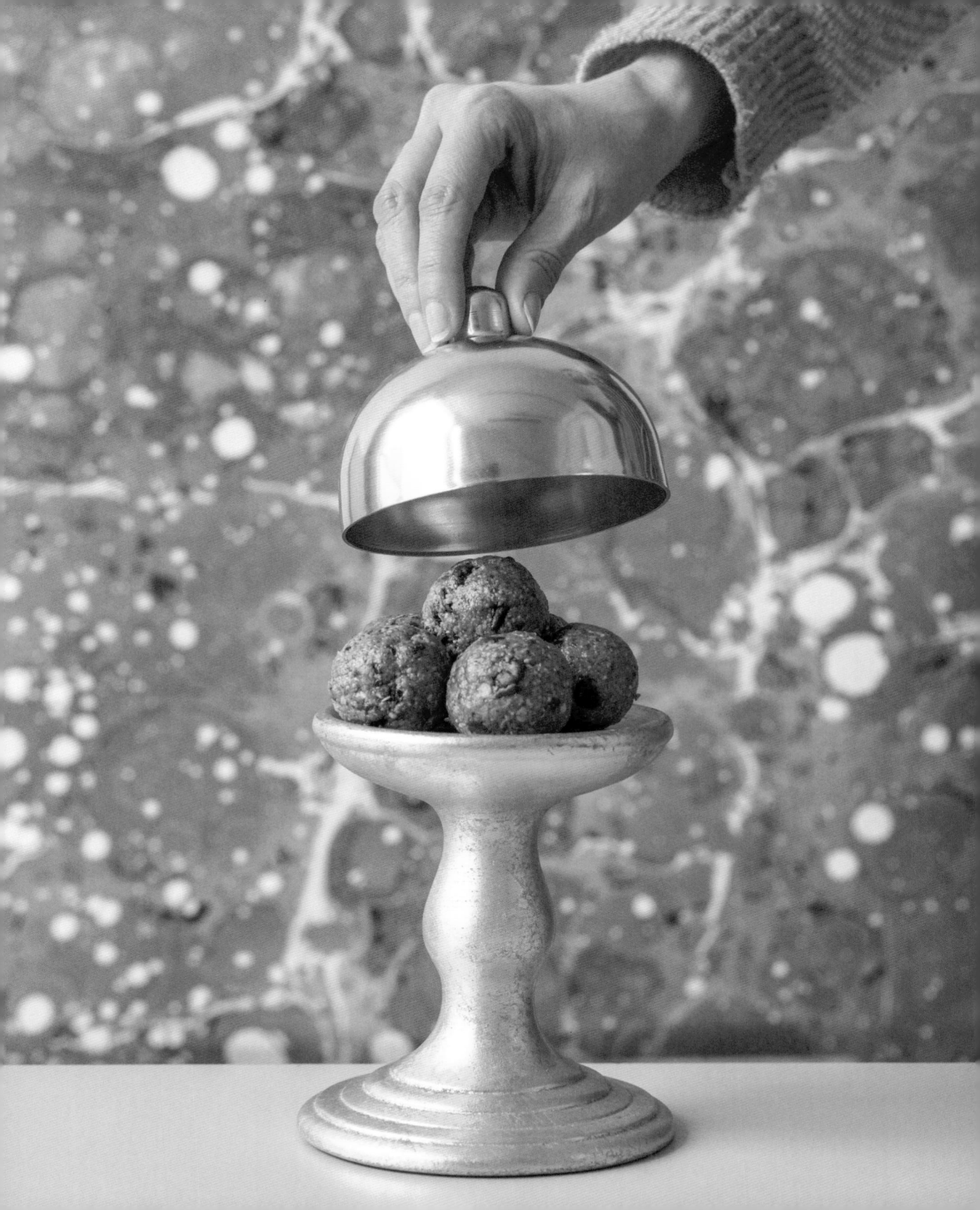

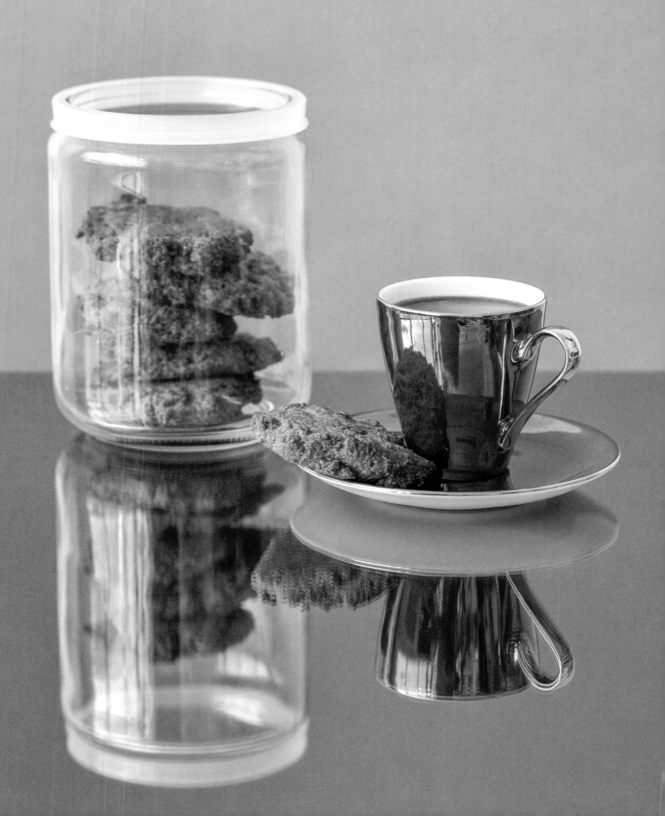

CBD PUMPKIN CHOC CHIP COOKIES

///////////

Using pumpkin or sweet potato purée as a baking ingredient adds moisture and subtle sweetness. Plus, they bring additional fibre and tons of vitamin A, making these cookies a treat you can really feel good about. I sometimes like to eat these slathered with peanut butter or almond butter on top.

2 tablespoons ground chia seeds
6 tablespoons water
85 g/½ cup coconut sugar
120 ml/½ cup melted coconut oil
1 teaspoon CBD oil
115 g/½ cup pumpkin or sweet potato purée
1 teaspoon bicarbonate of/ baking soda
1 teaspoon ground cinnamon
½ teaspoon ground cardamom
¼ teaspoon fine sea salt
190 g/2 cups almond flour
45 g/1½ oz. vegan dark/bittersweet chocolate, roughly chopped

baking sheet, lined with baking parchment

MAKES 12/3 COOKIES PER SERVING

Preheat the oven to 180°C (350°F) Gas 4.

Mix together the ground chia seeds and water in a large bowl and leave to stand for 5–10 minutes until gelatinous in texture.

Add the coconut sugar, melted coconut oil, CBD oil and pumpkin or sweet potato purée and mix well to combine. Add the bicarbonate of/ baking soda and stir well. Add the cinnamon, cardamom and salt and stir to incorporate. Mix in the almond flour until fully incorporated. You should have a slightly wet but pretty cohesive dough. Finally, fold in the chopped chocolate.

Divide the dough into roughly 12 small portions and then roll each one into a ball. Place the balls onto the prepared baking sheet and flatten each one slightly. Bake in the preheated oven for about 12–14 minutes until the cookies are golden. Let them cool completely on the baking sheet before transferring to a serving plate or container.

The cookies will keep, refrigerated, for up to 1 week.

CBD RASPBERRY & BANANA NICE CREAM

///////////////

'Nice' cream couldn't be easier to make. All you really need are frozen bananas and a food processor, but this version is made a little more exciting with a raspberry ripple (and CBD, of course).

3 frozen bananas, peeled and
    chopped
1 teaspoon vanilla extract
½ teaspoon CBD oil
2 tablespoons plus 60ml/¼ cup
    full-fat coconut milk
125 g/1 cup frozen raspberries

SERVES 2

In a food processor or blender, process the bananas, vanilla, CBD oil and the 2 tablespoons of coconut milk together until you have a smooth mixture. Pour into a freezerproof container.

Put raspberries and remaining 60 ml/¼ cup of the coconut milk into the food processor or blender and process until smooth. Pour the raspberry mixture on top of the banana mixture in the container and drag a small rubber spatula or knife gently through to create ripples of the raspberry in the banana. Pop into the freezer for about 10 minutes to firm up before serving.

You can store the nice cream in the freezer, but let it thaw for about 10–15 minutes before serving if it has been in there for a while. It will keep for 1–2 weeks.

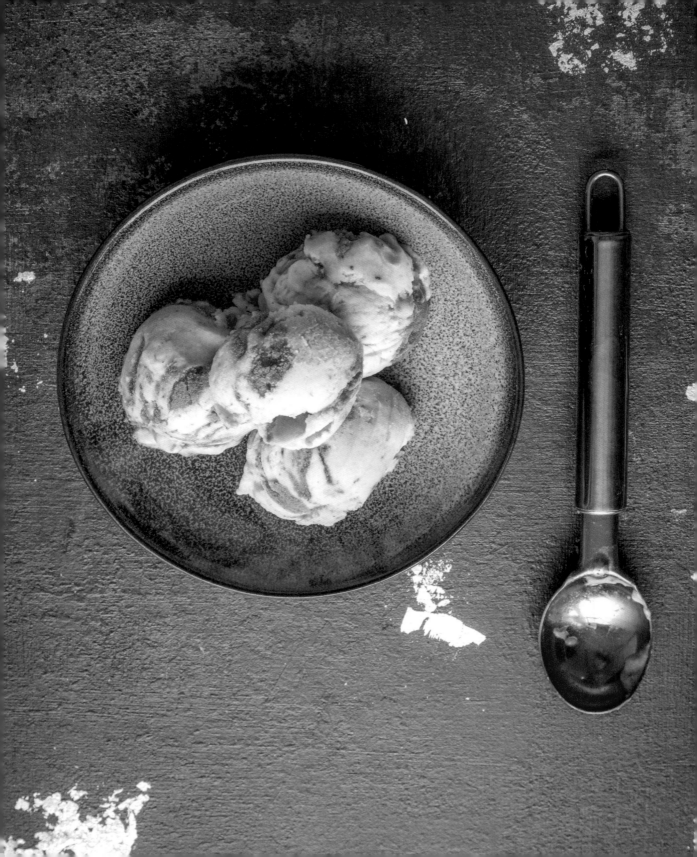

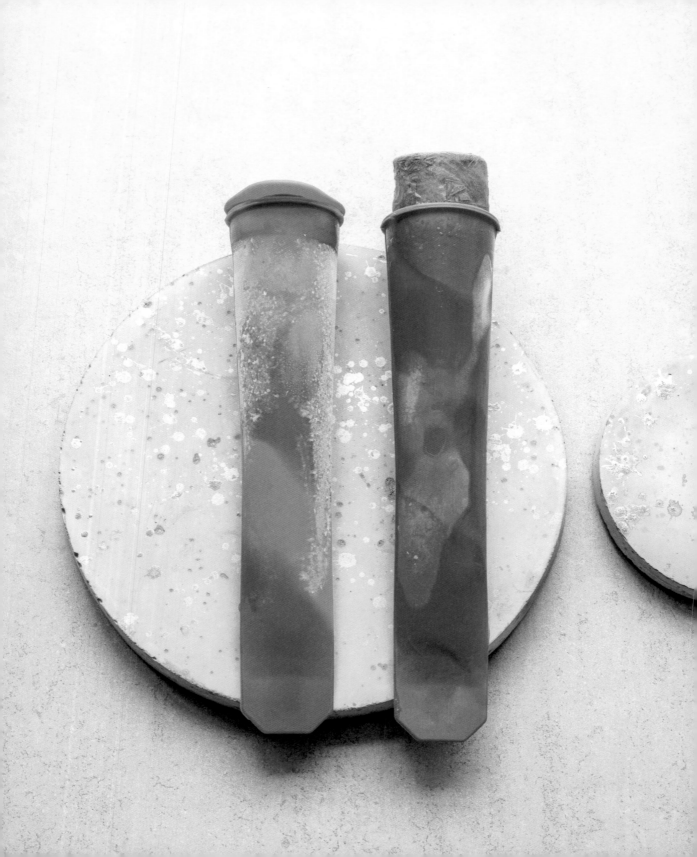

CBD REISHI CACAO CASHEW FUDGESICLES

Cashews make an amazing neutral nut milk when blended with water that, unlike many, you can use straight away because it doesn't need straining. The creaminess is perfect for making this simple, healthed-up version of fudgesicle pops.

120 g/1 cup raw cashews, soaked for an hour or overnight
475 ml/2 cups filtered water
2 tablespoons cacao powder
2 tablespoons maple syrup
2 teaspoons reishi mushroom powder
1 teaspoon CBD oil
pinch of sea salt

6-7 popsicle moulds

MAKES 6-7/1 PER SERVING

Combine all the ingredients in a blender and process until completely smooth. Pour into your popsicle moulds, then freeze until set (overnight is best).

Remove from the freezer a few minutes before serving.

Tip If you are having trouble getting the pops out, dunk the moulds very quickly into hot water.

CBD
CHOCOLATE
PUDDING

I used to be opposed to the concept of avocado chocolate pudding – until I actually tried it. When I finally decided to make a version for myself, I realized how silly I'd been to deprive myself for this long. A sweet treat that is packed with fibre and healthy fats, while still tasting nostalgically chocolaty? Sign me up. I like to portion this between 4 small jars and sometimes serve it topped with a little whipped coconut cream.

1 ripe avocado, peeled and pitted
1 banana, peeled and chopped
50 g/½ cup cacao powder
75 g/⅓ cup natural (no added sugar) smooth almond butter or peanut butter
60 ml/¼ cup maple syrup
1 teaspoon CBD oil
¼ teaspoon sea salt
whipped coconut cream, to serve (optional)

4 small jars or serving glasses

SERVES 4

Place all the ingredients in a food processor or blender and process until completely smooth. Divide the pudding between your small jars or serving glasses. Cover with the jar lids or clingfilm/plastic wrap and chill in the refrigerator for 1–2 hours before serving, topped with a little whipped coconut cream, if desired.

These little puddings will keep in the refrigerator for 1–2 days, but really the fresher the better.

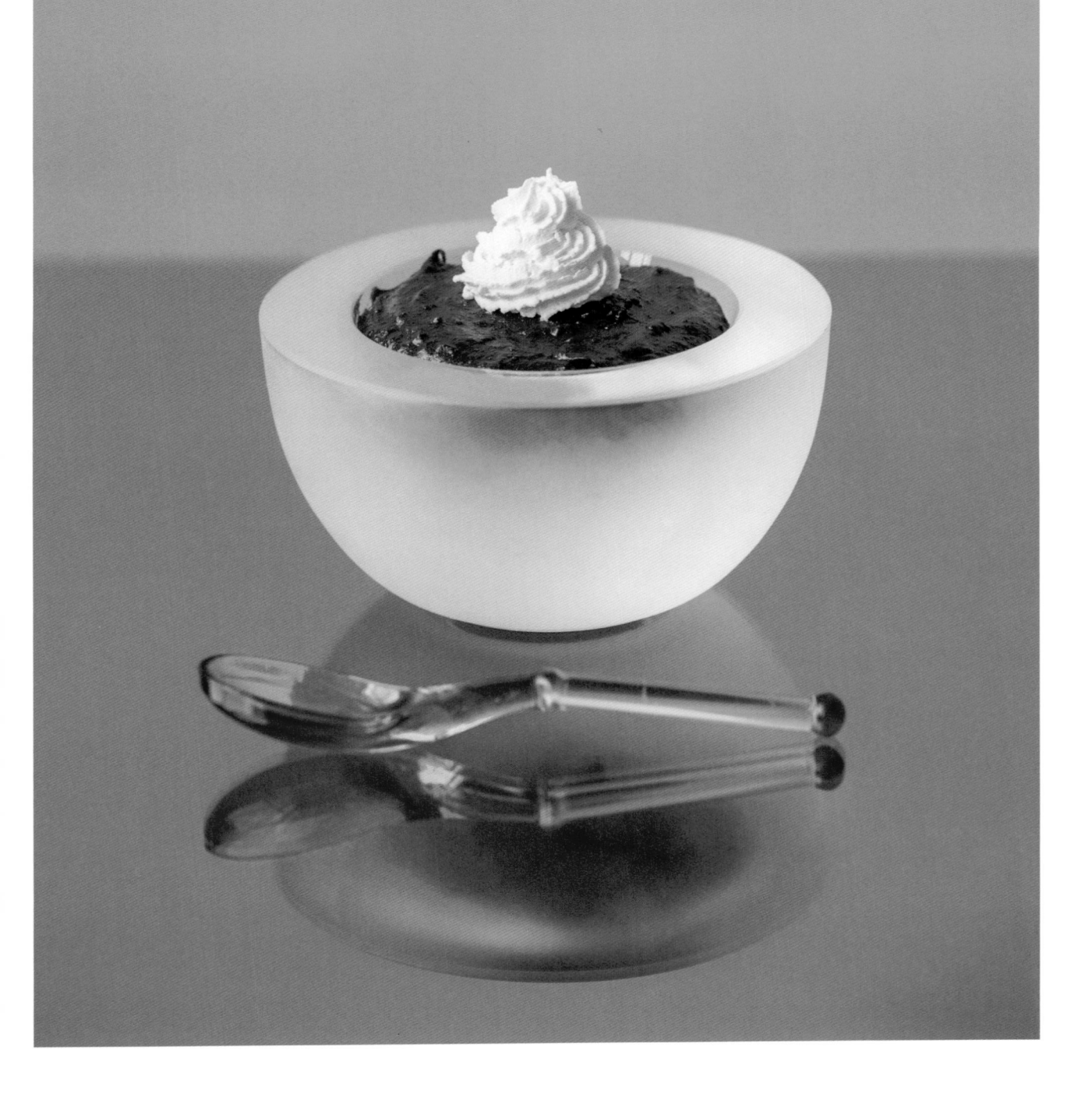

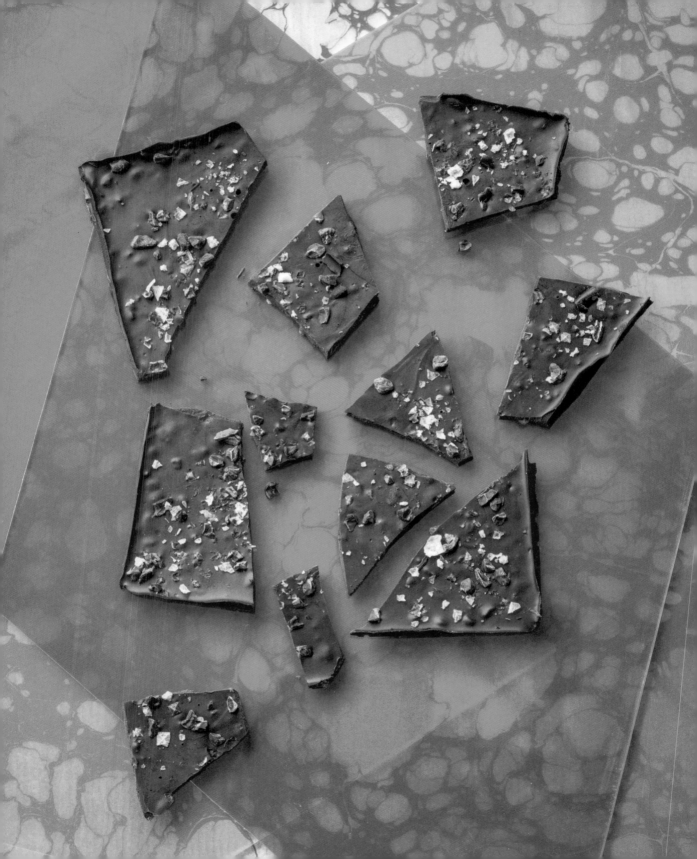

CBD SEA SALT & CACAO NIB CHOCOLATE BARK

//////////////

I love to create my own chocolate bars in the form of an easy chocolate bark. I've kept this one simple with cacao nibs for crunch and a little salty-sweet action from flaky sea salt. But feel free to add toasted nuts, dried fruit, toasted coconut – whatever sounds delicious to you!

100 g/3½ oz. vegan dark/
    bittersweet chocolate,
    roughly chopped
1 teaspoon CBD oil
2 tablespoons cacao nibs, divided
¾ teaspoon flaked sea salt, divided

*medium rectangular container,
lined with baking parchment
(I used 10 x 18-cm/4 x 7-inches)*

MAKES 4 SERVINGS

Put the chocolate into a large stainless steel or heatproof glass bowl set over a pan containing about 5–7.5 cm/2–3 inches boiling water. Make sure the base of the bowl does not touch the water. Stir with a rubber spatula occasionally until the chocolate has melted, then remove from the heat. Stir in the CBD oil immediately and mix until smooth. Add half the cacao nibs and half the sea salt and stir until evenly distributed.

Pour the chocolate into your prepared container, smoothing it into an even layer with the rubber spatula. Sprinkle with the remaining cacao nibs and sea salt and when cool enough, refrigerate for 1 hour or until set.

Break apart the set chocolate bark with your hands and serve. The bark will keep refrigerated in an airtight container for up to 1 month.

CBD DATE CARAMELS

So, there's no actual caramel-making involved here, which is very appealing to someone like me who finds boiling sugar slightly terrifying to handle. I use big Medjool dates, which have a naturally caramel-like flavour on their own. Dipped in melted chocolate, these look fancy but the ingredients list is short. I put a relatively small about of CBD oil in these (about half a dose per caramel), so I can enjoy a couple at a time.

12 Medjool dates, pitted
2 tablespoons natural (no added sugar) almond butter
1 teaspoon CBD oil
¼ teaspoon fine sea salt
1-2 teaspoons water, if needed
100 g/3½ oz. vegan dark/ bittersweet chocolate, chopped into small chunks
flaked sea salt, for topping (optional)

large plate, lined with baking parchment

MAKES 10–12/2 CARAMELS PER SERVING

In a food processor or high-speed blender, combine the dates, almond butter, CBD oil and salt and pulse to break the dates up and mix the ingredients. Add the water, as needed, to bring things together. (I used 2 teaspoons the first time I made this and 1 the second, so it depends on your dates and the consistency of your peanut butter.) Process on a medium speed until a sticky, fairly smooth dough forms. Break off a piece of the dough and roll it into a bite-size ball (just smaller than a ping-pong ball). Flatten the ball with your palms and squish the sides to make a square. Repeat with the rest of the date dough, placing the squares on your prepared plate as you make each one. Pop the squares into the freezer for 30 minutes to firm up or refrigerate overnight.

When you're ready, put the chocolate into a large stainless steel or heatproof glass bowl set over a pan containing about 5–7.5 cm/2–3 inches of boiling water. Make sure the base of the bowl does not touch the water. Stir with a rubber spatula occasionally until the chocolate has melted, then remove from the heat.

Take the date caramels out of the freezer/fridge and dunk them, one at a time, into the melted chocolate. Flip over with a rubber spatula to coat in a thin layer of chocolate on all sides, then use a fork to place them back onto the lined plate. Top with a small sprinkle of sea salt, if you like. Repeat with the remaining squares, then freeze for 30 minutes to set.

The date caramels will keep for 2–3 weeks in the refrigerator.

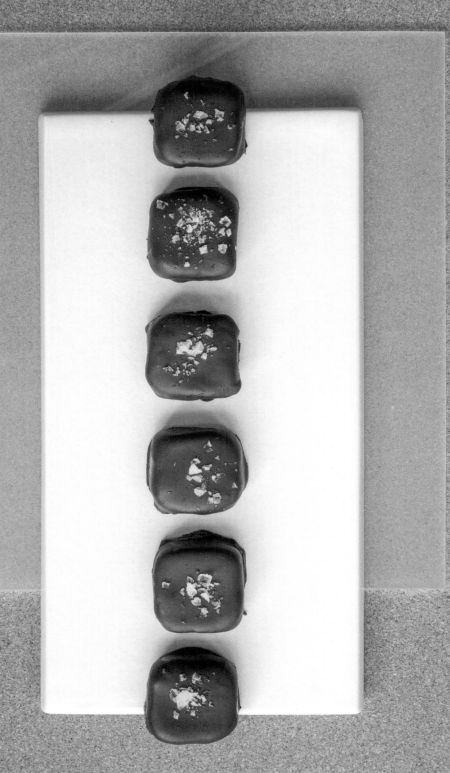

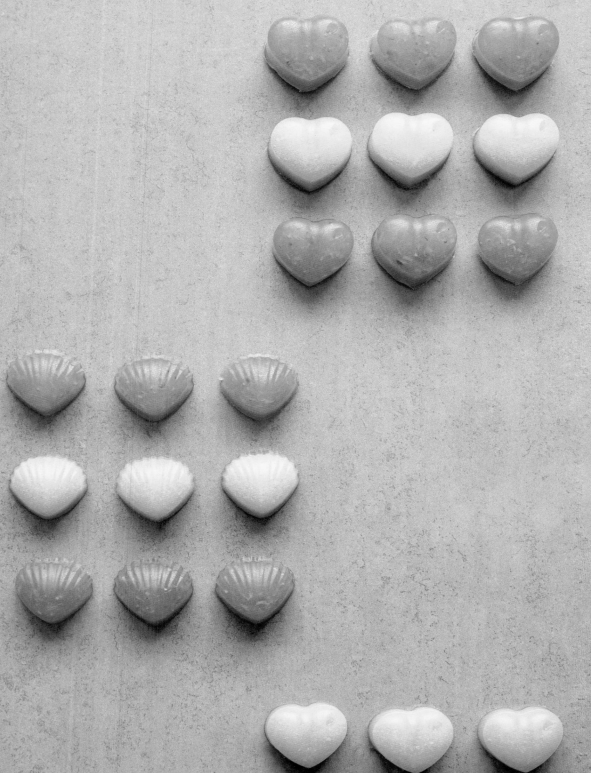

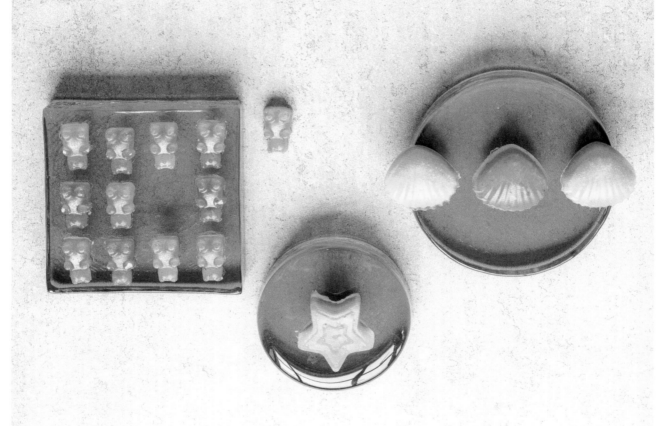

CBD MANGO GUMMIES

▰▰▰▰▰▰▰▰▰▰

Try these sunshiney mango gummies for a bonus hit of vitamins A and C. Vegan jel is a great plant-based alternative to gelatine, just make sure to get the unflavoured variety. I buy mine online.

300 g/1 scant cup peeled and pitted mango flesh, cut into small chunks
60 ml/¼ cup water
1 tablespoon freshly squeezed lemon juice
1½ tablespoons agave syrup
3 teaspoons CBD oil
3 tablespoons vegan jel

silicone candy moulds
squeeze dropper (most moulds come with a dropper)

MAKES 50–90 GUMMIES, DEPENDING ON THE MOULD SIZE/5–10 GUMMIES PER SERVING

Blend the mango chunks to a purée in a blender or food processor.

Combine the mango purée, water, lemon juice, agave syrup and CBD oil in a saucepan over a low heat and whisk until well-combined. When you see the mixture just start to bubble at the edges, turn off the heat and whisk in the jel.

Using the squeeze dropper, transfer the mixture into your gummy moulds. Leave to cool to room temperature and then refrigerate for 20 minutes until set.

Remove the gummies from their moulds and keep refrigerated in an airtight container for up to 1 month.

CBD BERRY GUMMIES

///////////

Surprisingly easy to make, these CBD gummies use real fruit, are sweetened with agave syrup and cost a fraction of the store-bought candies you might find elsewhere.

100 g/¾ cup fresh trimmed
   strawberries or raspberries
60 ml/¼ cup water
1 tablespoon freshly squeezed
   lemon juice
1½ tablespoons agave syrup
3 teaspoons CBD oil
3 tablespoons vegan jel

silicone candy moulds
squeeze dropper (most moulds
come with a dropper)

MAKES 50–90 GUMMIES, DEPENDING ON THE
MOULD SIZE/5–10 GUMMIES PER SERVING

Blend the strawberries or raspberries to a purée in a blender or food processor.

Combine the berry purée, water, lemon juice, agave syrup and CBD oil in a saucepan over a low heat and whisk until well combined. When you see the mixture just start to bubble at the edges, turn off the heat and whisk in the jel.

Using the squeeze dropper, transfer the mixture into your gummy moulds. Leave to cool to room temperature and then refrigerate for 20 minutes until set.

Remove the gummies from their moulds and keep refrigerated in an airtight container for up to 1 month.

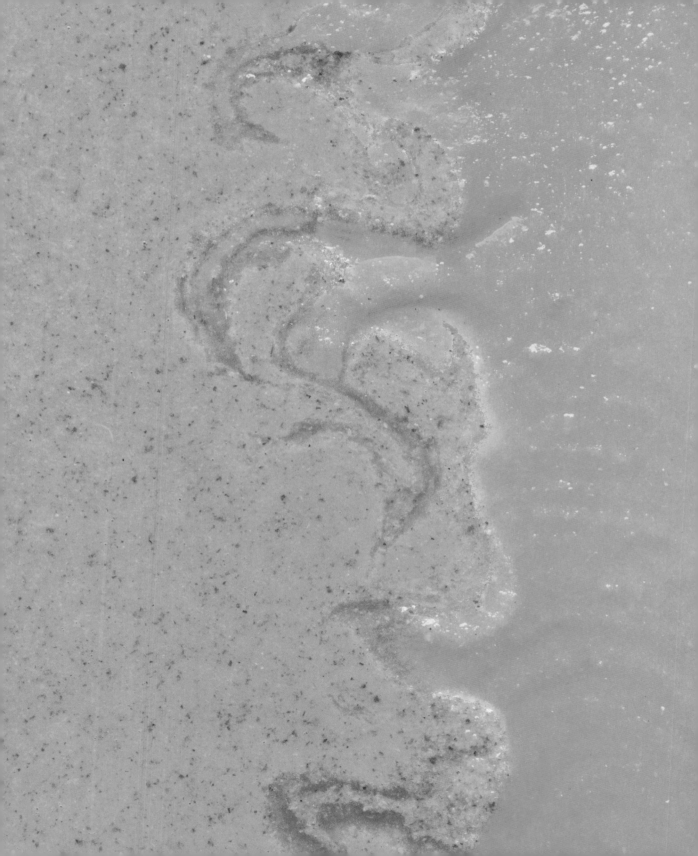

SAVOURIES

Combine CBD into your daily routine with these easy, delicious recipes.

TOMATO & BUTTERNUT SOUP
WITH CBD PESTO

///////////////

Butternut squash makes this soup creamy without any cream (or faux cream, for that matter) and a cozy blend of spicy, sweet and acidic. The roasted garlic can be prepared ahead of time, if needed.

olive oil, for drizzling and frying
1 head of garlic, skin-on but woody base sliced off
1 small red onion, finely chopped
½ teaspoon chilli flakes/hot red pepper flakes
500 g/4 heaped cups peeled butternut squash chopped into 2.5-cm/1-inch cubes
400-g/14-oz. can of crushed tomatoes
710 ml/3 cups water
salt and freshly ground black pepper

PESTO
60 g/2 cups fresh basil
2 roasted garlic cloves (from head of garlic above)
75 ml/⅓ cup olive oil
½ teaspoon CBD oil
2 tablespoons roasted unsalted cashews
freshly squeezed juice of ½ lemon
salt, to taste

SERVES 4

Preheat the oven to 200°C (400°F) Gas 6.

Drizzle a little olive oil on a small square of foil and place the head of garlic, cut-side down on the olive oil and wrap it in the foil. Roast in the preheated oven for 40 minutes until tender and fragrant. Let cool completely before handling. Remove the roasted cloves from their papery skins and set aside, separating out two cloves for the pesto.

In a large saucepan, heat about 2 tablespoons of olive oil over a medium heat. Add the red onion and sauté for about 5 minutes until softened. Add the chilli flakes/hot red pepper flakes, roasted garlic cloves, 1 teaspoon salt and the butternut squash cubes and stir to coat everything in the oil. Cook for about 3–4 minutes, stirring often. Add the canned tomatoes and water and bring to the boil. Turn down the heat and simmer, covered, for 20 minutes, stirring occasionally, until the butternut squash is tender and easily pierced with a fork. Remove from the heat. Purée the soup with an immersion blender or in a regular blender until smooth. Taste and adjust the seasoning to your liking.

While the soup is cooking, make the pesto by combining all the ingredients in a small food processor and processing until all the ingredients are chopped and well combined into a smooth pesto. Return the blended soup to the saucepan to heat through and serve hot, topped with a swirl of pesto. The soup and pesto will keep separately in the refrigerator for up to 1 week.

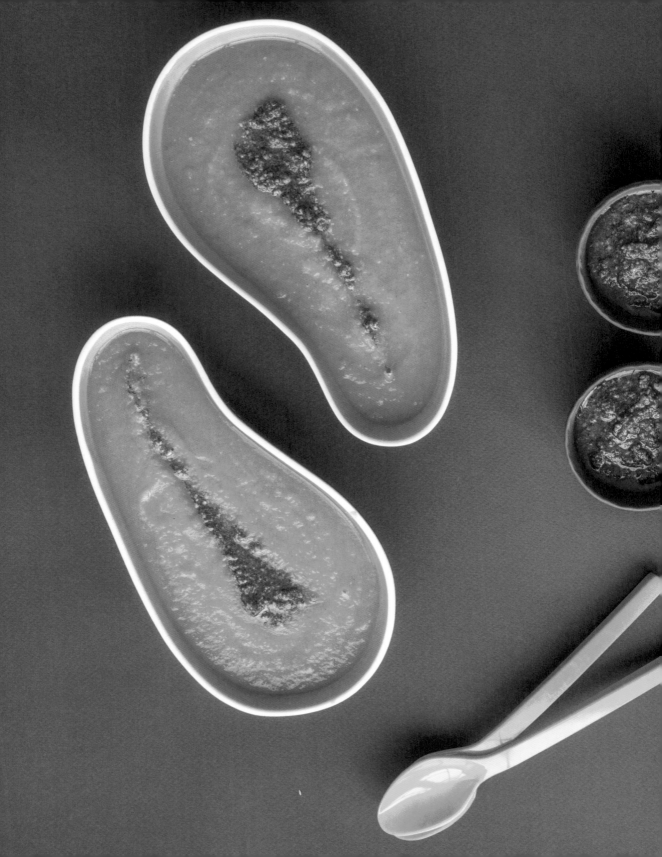

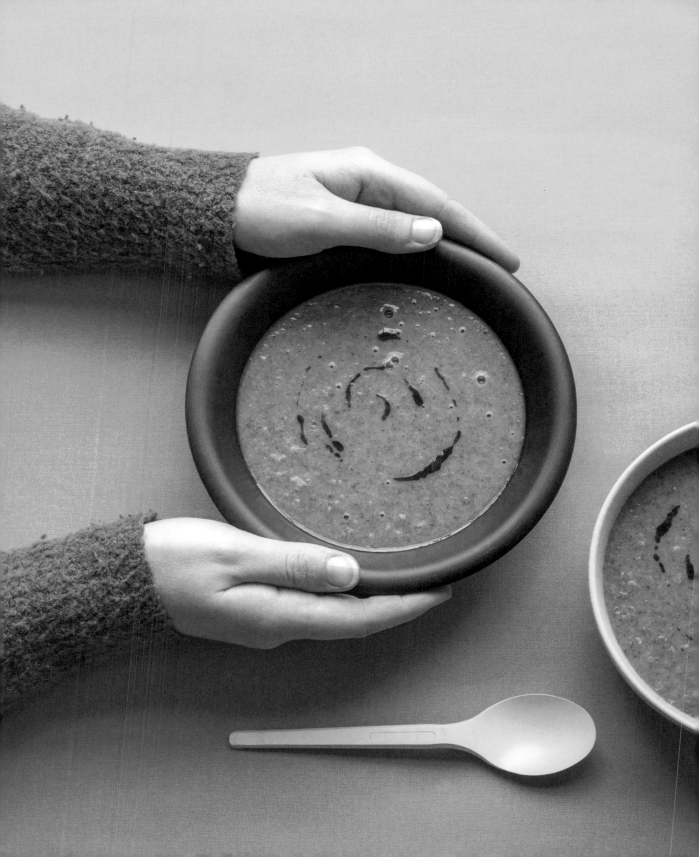

CBD LEEK & COURGETTE SOUP

Make this hearty, healthy vegetable soup for an extra dose of greens. It comes together quickly – so as to not let any of the ingredients get too mushy or lose their vibrant green colour. Add a little more texture and substance to it by stirring in cooked rice, quinoa or chickpeas or serve with some crusty bread on the side.

2 tablespoons olive oil
1 garlic clove, peeled and finely chopped
2 medium leeks, trimmed and thinly sliced
1 teaspoon salt
950 ml/4 cups vegetable stock
185 g/1½ cups frozen peas, thawed
2 medium courgettes/zucchini, chopped into 2.5-cm/1-inch pieces
10 leaves of curly kale, stems removed
30 g/½ packed cup fresh parsley, leaves only
30 g/½ packed cup fresh basil, leaves only
¼ teaspoon CBD oil per bowl, to serve
crusty bread or cooked rice, quinoa or chickpeas, to serve (optional)

SERVES 4–6

Heat the oil in a large saucepan over a medium heat. Add the garlic, leeks and salt and cook, stirring, for about 10 minutes until softened. Add the stock and bring to the boil. Add the peas and courgettes/zucchini and simmer, covered, for 3 minutes. Stir in the kale and simmer, covered, for another 2 minutes until the courgettes/zucchini are tender.

Remove the soup from the heat and stir in the parsley and basil. Let cool, uncovered, for 5 minutes and then purée with an immersion blender or in a regular blender in batches until smooth.

Return the blended soup to the pan and warm through over a low heat to serve. Pour into individual bowls and stir the ¼ teaspoon CBD oil into each. Serve with the accompaniments of your choosing. The soup will keep in the refrigerator for up to 1 week.

CBD AVOCADO TOAST

////////////////

I should really stop giving people recipes for avocado toast. BUT, I love the simple trick of putting the CBD oil on freshly toasted bread before the avocado. It goes by completely undetected and makes a great breakfast.

1 large or 2 small slices of bread
(I like sourdough or sprouted)
1 garlic clove, sliced in half
¼ teaspoon CBD oil
½ avocado, pitted
generous pinch of sea salt
pinch of freshly ground black
    pepper
pinch of chilli flakes/hot red
    pepper flakes
1 tablespoon freshly chopped
    coriander/cilantro, parsley
    or basil (or a combo)
sprinkle of vegan feta, to finish
    (optional)

SERVES 1

Toast the bread to your liking. While it is still hot, rub the garlic clove halves, cut-side down, onto your toast. Drizzle the toast evenly with CBD oil.

Scoop the avocado flesh from its skin and lightly smush it onto the toast with a fork or knife. Sprinkle with the salt, pepper, chilli flakes/hot red pepper flakes, fresh herb(s) and vegan feta (if using). Enjoy immediately.

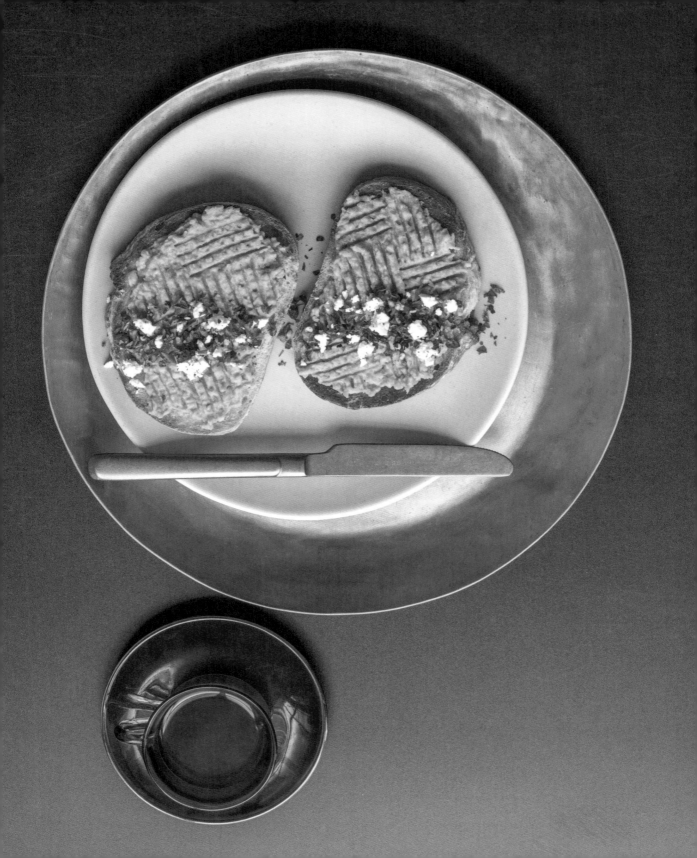

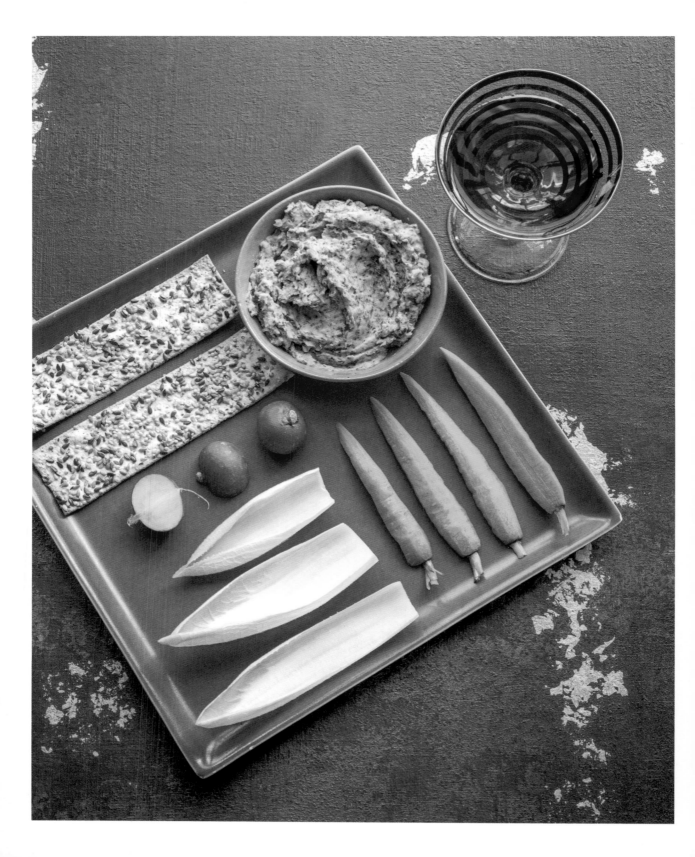

CBD HERBY WHITE BEAN & GARLIC DIP

This purée is a great dip with crudité vegetables such as sliced raw carrot, radish or chicory/endive leaves, crackers or sliced baguette. It even makes a flavourful spread for sandwiches. Plenty of fresh herbs and a little lemon juice give it a vibrant freshness.

2 tablespoons olive oil, plus extra to serve
2 small garlic cloves, peeled and roughly chopped
400-g/14-oz. can of cooked white beans (such as cannellini or haricot/navy beans), drained and rinsed
15 g/¼ packed cup fresh parsley leaves
15 g/¼ packed cup fresh coriander/cilantro leaves
2 tablespoons freshly snipped chives
freshly squeezed juice of ½ lemon
½ teaspoon CBD oil
sea salt

SERVES 4

In a medium frying pan/skillet, heat the olive oil over a low-medium heat. Add the garlic and cook for 1–2 minutes until fragrant but not browning. Add the white beans and cook, stirring, for another 2 minutes.

Transfer the garlic beans to a food processor or blender. Add the remaining ingredients, seasoning to taste with the salt, and process until the ingredients are combined and smooth, scraping down the sides once or twice to make sure everything is incorporated.

Transfer the dip to a bowl and either serve as it is or refrigerate until you're ready to serve.

GRILLED LETTUCE, CHICKPEA & RADISH SALAD WITH MISO & GARLIC CBD VINAIGRETTE

//////////////////

This is a great hearty salad with protein from the chickpeas, green leaves, peppery radishes and lots of umami flavour from the dressing.

avocado or olive oil, for brushing
    and frying
1 head of romaine/cos lettuce,
    washed, dried, trimmed and
    split down the middle
    lengthways
400-g/14-oz. can of cooked
    chickpeas, drained and rinsed
pinch of cayenne pepper
3 radishes, thinly sliced

MISO & GARLIC CBD VINAIGRETTE
4 tablespoons avocado or olive oil
freshly squeezed juice of ½ lemon
2 teaspoons light miso paste
1 teaspoon Dijon mustard
1 garlic clove, finely chopped
    or grated on a microplane
salt and cracked black pepper,
    to taste
½ teaspoon CBD oil

SERVES 2

To make the salad dressing, whisk all the ingredients together in a medium bowl or jar until combined. Set aside.

Brush the cut inside of the romaine/cos lettuce with avocado or olive oil and sprinkle with salt. Heat a cast-iron frying pan/skillet over a medium-high heat. Once the pan/skillet is hot, place the lettuce halves oiled-side down in the pan. Use a spatula to press the lettuce wedges into the hot pan, they should sizzle. Continue to cook for 3–4 minutes until the lettuce is charred and lightly wilted but still vibrantly green in parts. Remove from the pan/skillet and set aside.

Add a little more avocado or olive oil to the pan, keeping the heat at medium-high. Add the chickpeas with a generous pinch of salt and the cayenne pepper. Cook for about 3–5 minutes, stirring occasionally, until the chickpeas are heated through and golden in spots.

Serve the romaine/cos lettuce, grilled side up, scattered with chickpeas and sliced radishes, with the dressing drizzled on top.

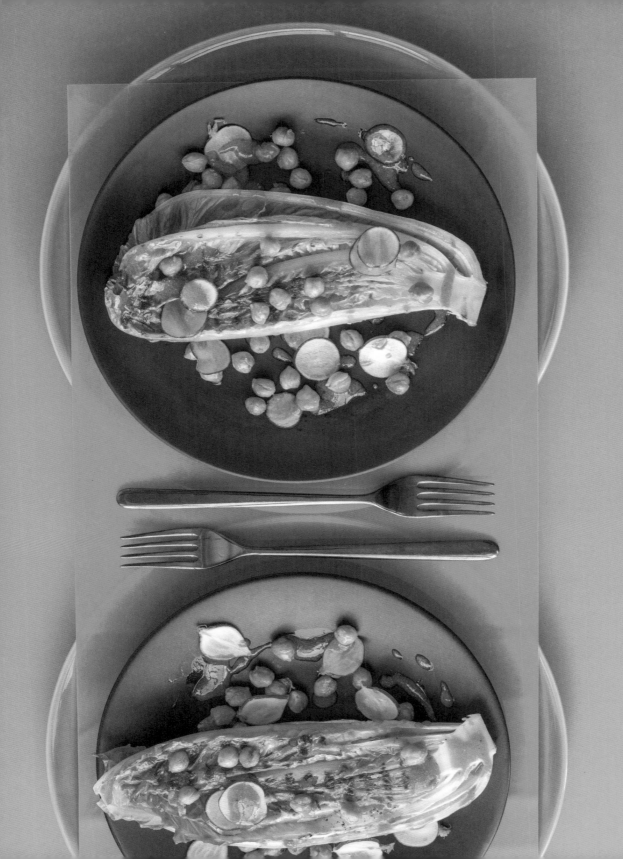

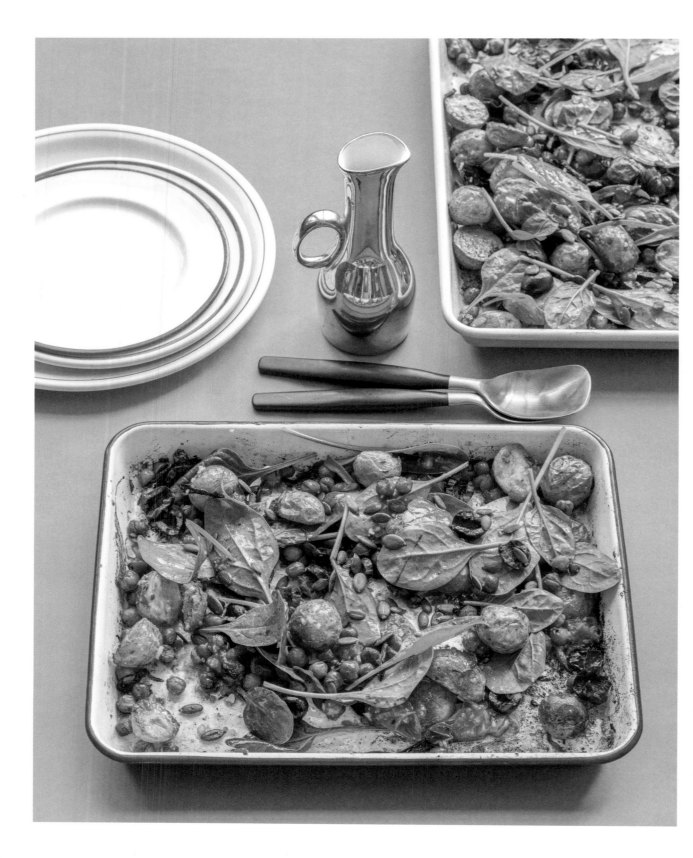

ROASTED POTATO & TOMATO BAKE WITH CBD OLIVE OIL, SHALLOT & LEMON DRESSING

I like to serve this as a meal as is, but it's great as a side dish too. You will have to use two baking dishes, but this is otherwise a pretty low-maintenance dinner.

450 g/1 lb. baby potatoes or fingerling potatoes, halved lengthways
350 g/12 oz. cherry or grape tomatoes, halved
400-g/14-oz. can of cooked chickpeas, drained and rinsed
½ small red onion, thinly sliced
1–2 tablespoons olive oil
generous pinch of salt
30 g/¼ cup Kalamata or black olives, pitted and torn
handful of baby spinach leaves or rocket/arugula, to serve
35 g/¼ cup toasted pumpkin seeds/pepitas, to serve

DRESSING
60 ml/¼ cup olive oil
freshly squeezed juice of 1 lemon
½ teaspoon CBD oil
2 tablespoons finely chopped shallot
1 teaspoon Dijon mustard
½ teaspoon sea salt
pinch of freshly ground black pepper

SERVES 4

Preheat the oven to 200°C (400°F) Gas 6.

In a large bowl, toss the potatoes, tomatoes, chickpeas and onion with the olive oil and salt. Spread the mixture out between two baking dishes in a single, even layer and roast in the preheated oven for 20 minutes. Rotate the dishes and continue to roast for another 10–15 minutes until the tomatoes have collapsed and the potatoes are golden.

Meanwhile, whisk together the dressing ingredients. Alternatively, you can blitz them together in a food processor to save time on finely chopping the shallot, if you like.

Drizzle the roasted potatoes and tomatoes with a few spoonfuls of the dressing and top with olives and baby spinach leaves or rocket/arugula. Toss to combine. Finish with a scattering of toasted pumpkin seeds/pepitas, taste for seasoning and serve.

I like to serve this right off the baking dishes with more dressing as desired.

LENTIL & SWEET POTATO BOWL
WITH CBD CHIMICHURRI

NNNNNNNNN

I love making this for lunches for the week ahead. But it's equally nice for a shared dinner. The chimichurri is great for livening up a bunch of other things like roasted vegetables and soups.

190 g/1 cup dry Puy lentils/French lentils
1 large sweet potato (or 2 small), peeled and cut into, 2.5-cm/ 1-inch cubes
2 tablespoons olive oil
1 bunch of kale, stems removed, roughly chopped
140 g/1 cup toasted walnuts, roughly chopped, to serve
salt and freshly ground black pepper

CHIMICHURRI
15 g/¼ packed cup fresh parsley
15 g/¼ packed cup fresh coriander/ cilantro
2 tablespoons finely chopped shallot
75 ml/⅓ cup olive oil
freshly squeezed juice of ½ lemon
1 teaspoon CBD oil
sea salt

SERVES 3–4

Preheat the oven to 190C (375°F) Gas 5.

In a saucepan, combine the lentils with 950 ml/ 4 cups water and a generous pinch of salt. Bring to the boil over a medium-high heat. Once boiling, turn the heat down and simmer, covered, for 25–30 minutes until the lentils are just tender. Drain and set aside.

Meanwhile, toss the sweet potato cubes with 1 tablespoon of the olive oil and a large pinch of salt in a bowl. Spread on a baking sheet and roast in the preheated oven for about 30 minutes, until golden and tender.

In another large bowl, combine the kale, the second tablespoon of olive oil and some salt and pepper. Use your hands to rub the olive oil into the kale, making sure the kale is well covered. Massage the kale for 20–30 seconds. This helps to break the leaves down, making them more tender. Set side.

Make the chimichurri by combining all the ingredients in a food processor or blender and processing until the herbs are finely chopped and the ingredients are evenly combined.

Toss a spoonful or two of the dressing into the cooked lentils and let sit until you're ready to serve.

Divide the kale between bowls and top each with lentils and sweet potato. Spoon over some chimichurri and top each bowl with toasted walnuts.

Store the elements separately in the refrigerator in airtight containers for up to 5 days. Bring to room temperature and/or reheat the lentils and sweet potato until hot all the way through before eating.

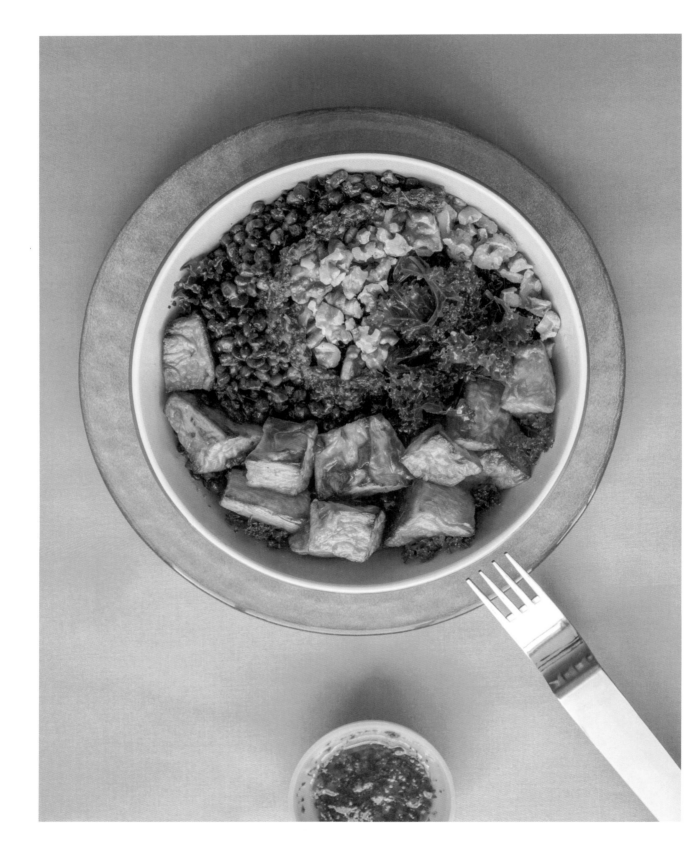

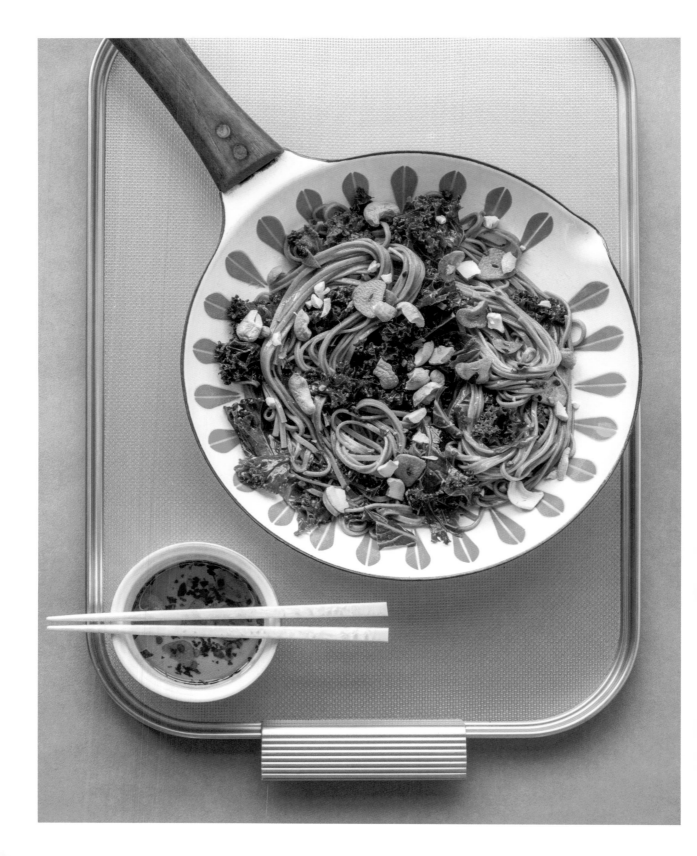

SOBA NOODLES, KALE & CASHEWS WITH CBD GARLIC & CHILLI OIL

I love this simple noodle dish served warm for an easy dinner or at room temperature the next day for lunch – I actually think the leftovers taste even better because the flavours have had more time to meld.

2 garlic cloves, peeled and finely chopped
1 teaspoon chilli flakes/hot red pepper flakes
60 ml/¼ cup avocado or olive oil
½ teaspoon CBD oil
60 g/½ cup raw cashews
225-g/8-oz. pack of buckwheat soba noodles
200 g/3 packed cups roughly chopped kale
salt

SERVES 2–3

Preheat the oven to 180°C (350°F) Gas 4.

In a medium frying pan/skillet, combine the garlic, chilli flakes/hot red pepper flakes and oil over a low heat. Heat through for about 4–5 minutes, giving a couple of stirs, until the garlic begins to sizzle and become fragrant, then remove from heat. Stir in the CBD oil and set aside until you're ready to use.

Spread the cashews out on a baking sheet and roast in the preheated oven for 8–10 minutes until golden.

Meanwhile, cook the noodles in salted boiling water for 1–2 minutes less than the package instructions state, adding the kale in the last 30 seconds of cooking. Drain the noodles and kale well and transfer to the pan with the garlic and chilli/chili oil. Toss to combine the ingredients and serve in portions scattered with the roasted cashews.

Refrigerate and store any leftovers in an airtight container for up to 5 days. Bring to room temperature or reheat until hot all the way through before serving.

GREEN CHICKPEA
CBD PANCAKES
///////////////

These chickpea/gram flour pancakes are on the slightly thicker, sturdier side of a savoury crepe. If you want to top these hearty, gluten-free pancakes with a sweet filling, simply leave out the herbs. You won't get the cool green colour, but you'll have nice golden pancakes for whatever tasty flavour combo you can think up.

125 g/1 cup chickpea/gram flour
295 ml/1¼ cups water
2 handfuls of fresh herbs such as parsley, basil and/or coriander/cilantro
½ teaspoon salt, or more to taste
¼–½ teaspoon CBD oil
olive oil, for frying

SAVOURY TOPPING IDEAS
sautéed mushrooms
roasted tomatoes
avocado
pesto

MAKES ABOUT 4 PANCAKES/SERVES 2

In a blender, combine the chickpea/gram flour with the water, herbs, salt and CBD oil and process until you get a smooth batter. Let the batter stand at room temperature for 10 minutes.

Heat the olive oil in a small non-stick frying pan/skillet over a medium heat. Add approximately 60–90 ml/¼–⅓ cup of the batter to the warm pan and swirl it around so that it covers the base of the pan. Cook for about 2–3 minutes, until the batter begins to form bubbles. Flip over with a spatula and cook for another 1–2 minutes on the other side until golden and cooked through. Remove to a plate and keep warm until ready to serve.

Repeat with the remaining batter – you may need to add a little more oil to the pan as you go. Serve the pancakes with your desired toppings.

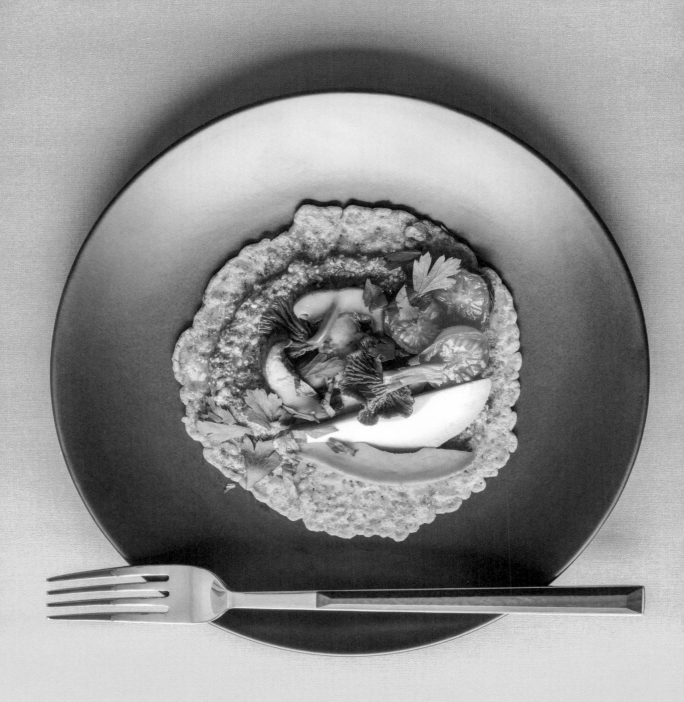

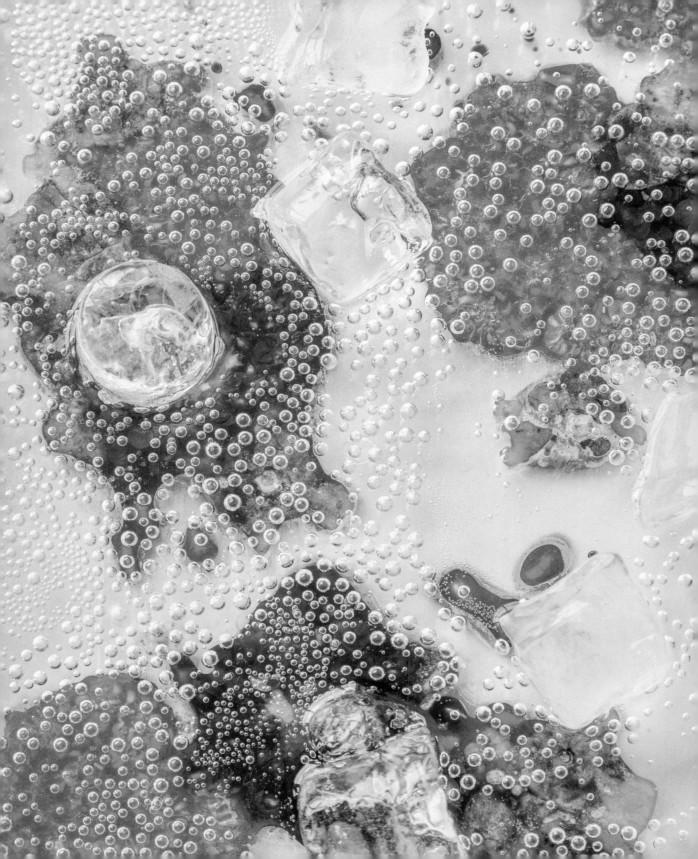

COCKTAILS & MOCKTAILS

A luxurious way to enjoy
your CBD dose, with or
without alcohol.

CBD GIN & BLACKBERRY BRAMBLE

░░░░░░░░░░░░

Muddled blackberries add beautiful colour and a fresh, fruity vibrancy to this cocktail.

60 g/½ cup fresh blackberries, plus extra to serve
60 ml/2 oz. gin
2 tablespoons agave syrup or simple sugar syrup
3 tablespoons freshly squeezed lemon juice
½ teaspoon CBD oil
club soda, to top up
ice cubes, to serve

medium jar with a lid or cocktail shaker

SERVES 2

In the jar with a lid or a cocktail shaker, combine the blackberries, gin, agave or sugar syrup, lemon juice and CBD oil and muddle the blackberries with the back of a spoon or a muddler until they have broken up and released their juices. Stir everything together and pour into ice-filled glasses through a fine-mesh sieve/strainer to remove the blackberry seeds. Top up with club soda and garnish with extra blackberries, to serve.

CBD TOM COLLINS

░░░░░░░░░░░░

This simple and classic cocktail gets even better with a little CBD oil. The extra lemon wedges to squeeze over and serve are a must for me.

60 ml/2 oz. gin
2 tablespoons agave syrup or simple sugar syrup
2 tablespoons freshly squeezed lemon juice
¼–½ teaspoon CBD oil
club soda, to top up
ice cubes, to serve
lemon wedges, to serve

medium jar with a lid or cocktail shaker

SERVES 2

Combine the gin, agave or sugar syrup, lemon juice and CBD oil in the jar or cocktail shaker with some ice. Shake well to combine. Strain the cocktail into two glasses over fresh ice. Top up each glass with club soda and serve with lemon wedges.

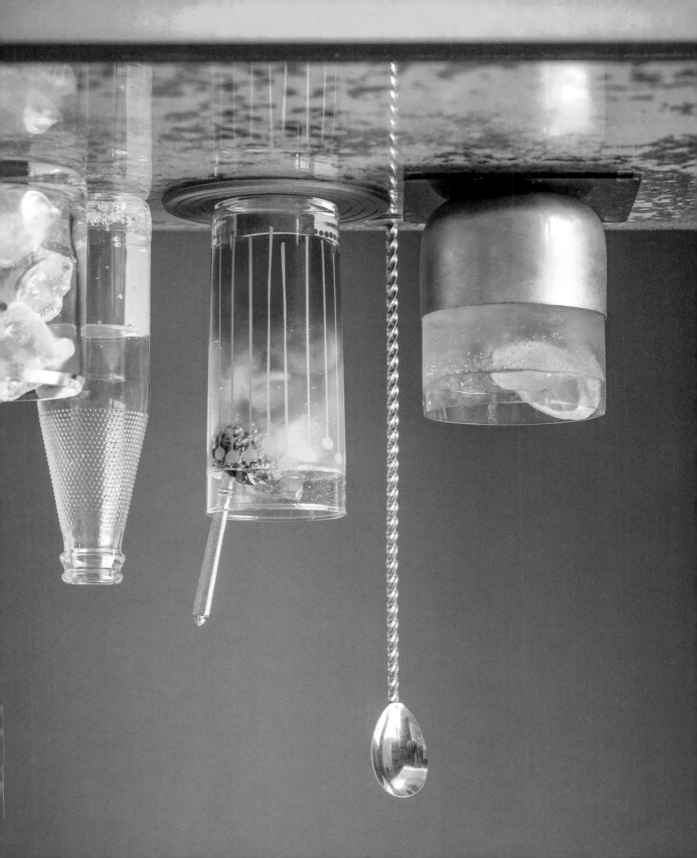

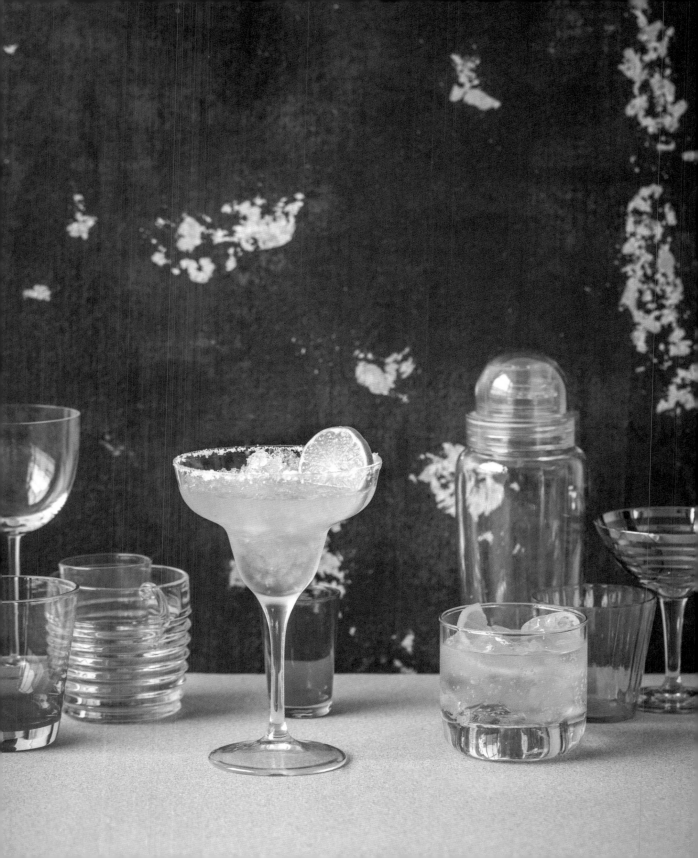

CBD ELDERFLOWER SPRITZ

Crisp sparkling wine and floral, sweet elderflower both mix well with the herbal notes of CBD. I love this cocktail at the beginning of the evening or as part of a long lunch.

2 tablespoons St. Germain or elderflower liqueur
¼ teaspoon CBD oil
60 ml/¼ cup Prosecco or cava
2 tablespoons club soda
ice cubes, to serve
lemon wedge, to serve

SERVES 1

Combine the St. Germain or elderflower liqueur with the CBD oil in a glass tumbler or wine glass and stir to combine. Fill the glass with ice and pour over the Prosecco or cava. Top with the club soda and serve with a wedge of lemon.

SIMPLE CBD MARGARITA

A strong, lime-forward margarita is the best kind in my opinion, but sometimes I like to cut this with some club soda to take the edge off.

60 ml/2 oz. tequila
30 ml/1 oz. freshly squeezed lime juice, plus a lime slice to serve
1 tablespoon agave syrup
¼ teaspoon CBD oil
sea salt, to serve (optional)
ice cubes, to serve

medium jar with a lid or cocktail shaker

SERVES 1

Wet the rim of a margarita glass and press into sea salt, if using, to garnish the rim. Combine the tequila, lime juice, agave syrup and CBD oil in the jar with a lid or cocktail shaker and shake to combine. Pour into the prepared glass (if using salt) over ice. Serve with a slice of lime.

CBD WATERMELON MOCKTAIL

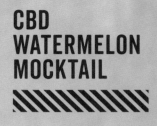

Refreshingly sweet watermelon is good enough on its own, but when blended with ice, lime juice and CBD, it makes for something special. This is an easy option for when you want a fun-looking drink without the booze.

900 g/6 cups peeled, deseeded and chopped watermelon flesh
6–8 ice cubes
freshly squeezed juice of ½ lime, the other half cut into wedges to serve
pinch of sea salt
1 teaspoon CBD oil

SERVES 4

Combine all the ingredients in a blender and process to a smooth purée. Serve immediately garnished with lime wedges.

CBD POMEGRANATE & KOMBUCHA MOCKTAIL

Kombucha, a kind of fermented tea, is one of my favourite alcohol alternatives (keep in mind that many brands do contain trace amounts of alcohol, but that's less than 0.5 per cent per bottle). It's got fizz and complex flavour and it packs in those natural probiotics for better gut health. Pomegranate brings a tangy-sweet flavour that makes this drink pop, but feel free to play around with other fruit juice mixers.

60 ml/¼ cup pomegranate juice
1 tablespoon freshly squeezed lemon juice
¼ teaspoon CBD oil
120 ml/½ cup plain kombucha
ice cubes, to serve
1 heaped teaspoon pomegranate seeds, to garnish

SERVES 1

In a medium-sized serving glass, combine the pomegranate juice, lemon juice and CBD oil and stir to combine. Fill the glass with ice and top up with the kombucha, giving everything another final stir. Garnish the drink with pomegranate seeds and enjoy.

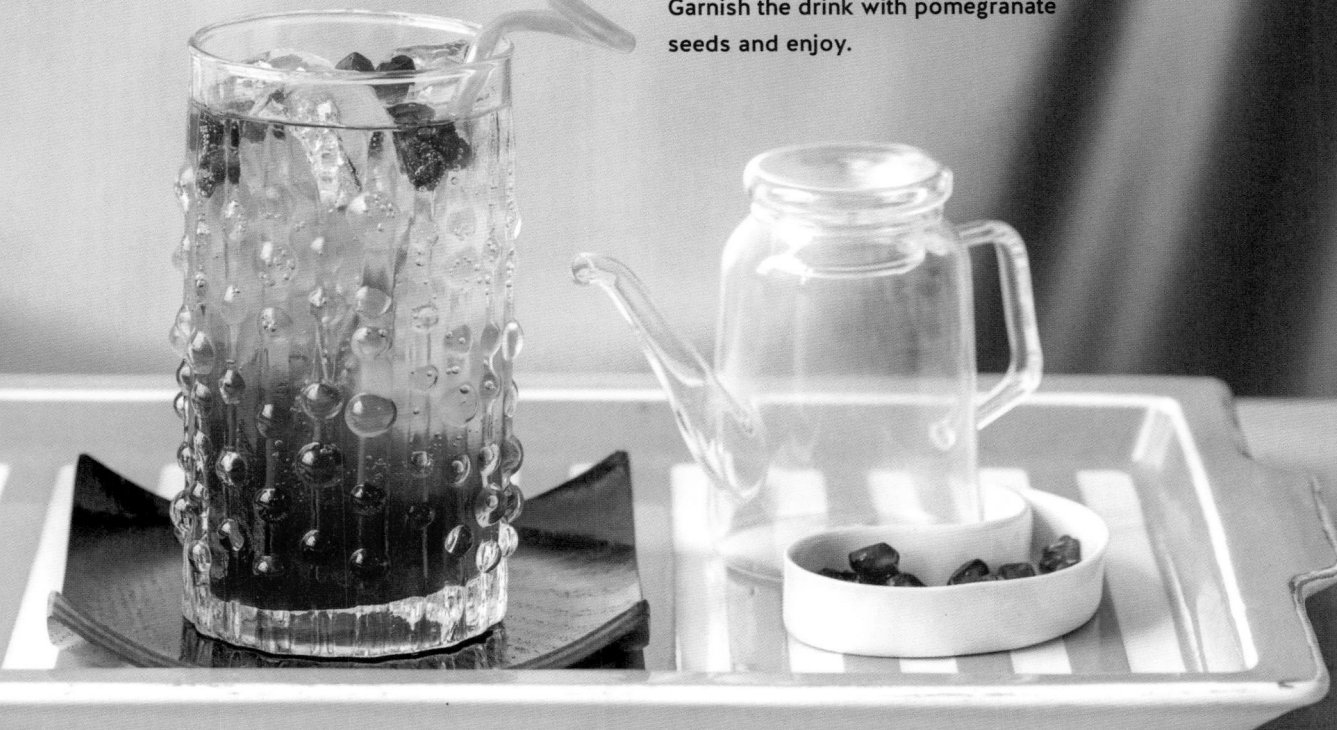

CBD GRAPEFRUIT & ROSE MOCKTAIL

A little sweet, a little sour and slightly floral, this mocktail is deceptively complex. The CBD makes it great for chilling out sans booze.

freshly squeezed juice of ½ large
    ruby red grapefruit, plus
    grapefruit slice to serve
    (about 120 ml/½ cup)
1 teaspoon rosewater
¼ teaspoon CBD oil
ice cubes, to serve
120 ml/½ cup club soda, to top up

jar with a lid

SERVES 1

Combine the grapefruit juice, rosewater and CBD oil in the jar, screw on the lid and shake to combine the ingredients. Pour into a glass over ice and top up with the club soda. Serve with a slice of grapefruit.

CBD GINGER & LIME MOCKTAIL

A little bit like a Moscow mule, this mocktail has plenty of flavour and is great for relaxing, calming stomach issues or squashing cold symptoms. For a cheat's version of this, combine a good-quality non-alcoholic ginger beer with CBD oil and lots of fresh lime.

5-cm/2-inch piece of fresh ginger,
    peeled
freshly squeezed juice of 1 lime,
    plus lime wedges to serve
1 tablespoon agave syrup
120 ml/½ cup water
½ teaspoon CBD oil
ice cubes, to serve
475–710 ml/2–3 cups club soda

jar with a lid

SERVES 2

Combine the ginger, lime, agave syrup and water in a blender and process on a high speed until smooth. Pour the mixture through a fine-mesh sieve/strainer into the jar. Add the CBD oil, screw on the lid and shake to combine the ingredients.

Pour 60 ml/¼ cup of the ginger CBD liquid each into two tall glasses. Top each drink up with club soda and stir to combine. Top the mocktails with a dash each of the remaining ginger liquid for a bigger flavour punch, if you like, and serve with fresh lime wedges.

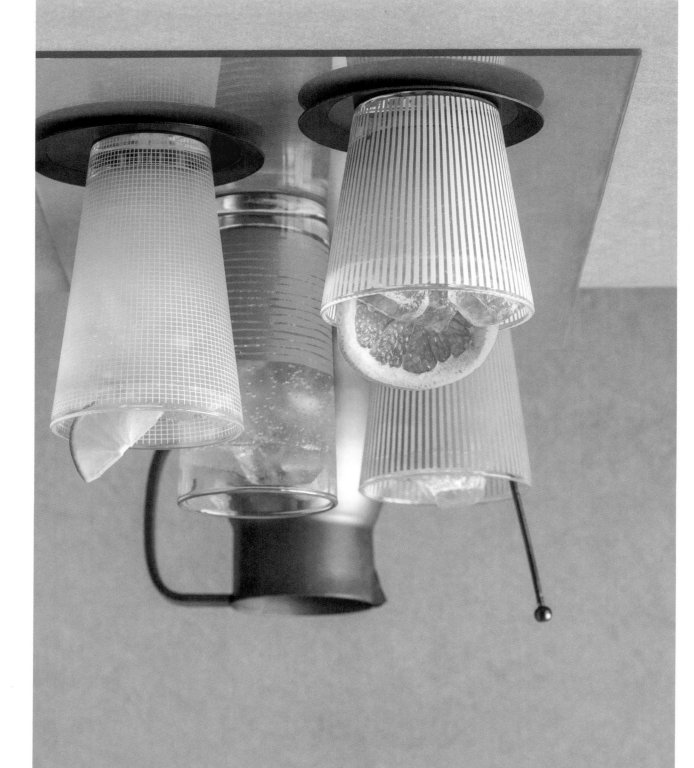

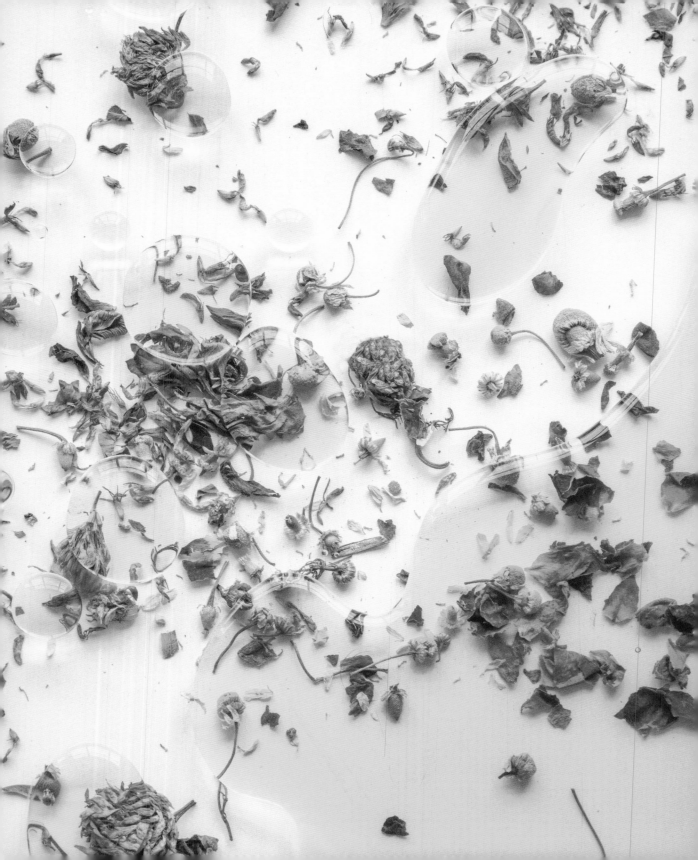

INFUSIONS

Drinks that combine
herbs with CBD for
super-powered benefits.

ANTI-ANXIETY CBD INFUSION

▧▧▧▧▧▧▧

Lemon balm is one of my favourite herbs for its ability to relieve anxiety and stress. Passionflower (despite its name) soothes and calms, as does friendly chamomile.

1 tablespoon dried passionflower stems and leaves

1 tablespoon dried lemon balm leaves

1 tablespoon dried chamomile flowers

1 litre/quart hot water (boiled and then cooled for about 2–5 minutes)

¼ teaspoon CBD oil and half a mug of just-boiled water per serving, to serve

1 litre/quart glass mason/kilner jar with a lid

MAKES 3–4 SERVINGS

Combine all the herbs and hot water in the mason/kilner jar. Mix so that the herbs are submerged in the water and place the lid on. Leave to infuse for a minimum of 4 hours or overnight at room temperature.

Strain the infusion and discard the herbs. Pour the liquid into a clean jar, or rinse out and use the same jar again. The infusion will keep at room temperature for 2–3 days or refrigerated for up to 1 week.

Serve the infusion warm by combining half a mug of the infusion with half a mug of just-boiled water. Stir ¼ teaspoon CBD oil into the warm liquid and enjoy.

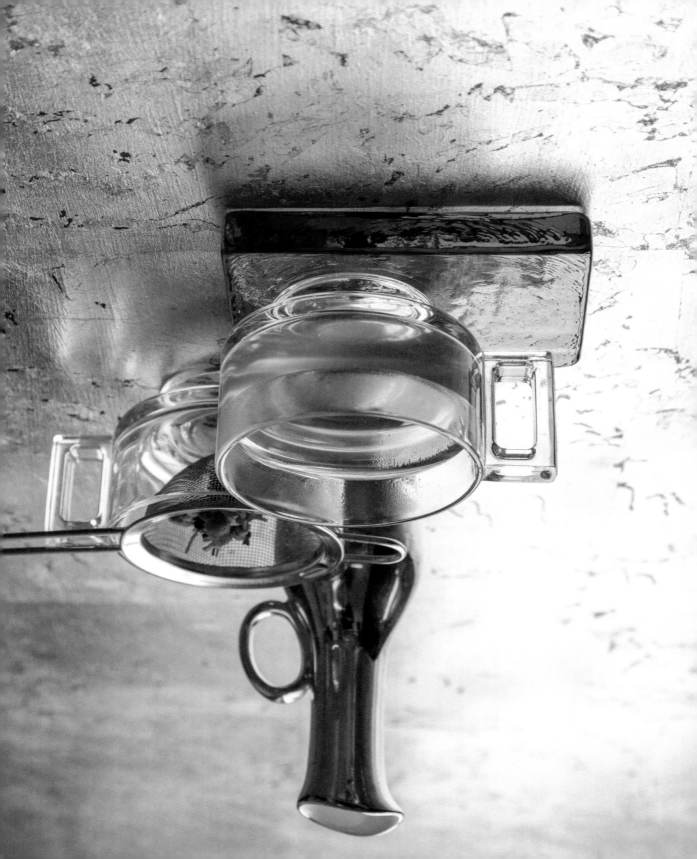

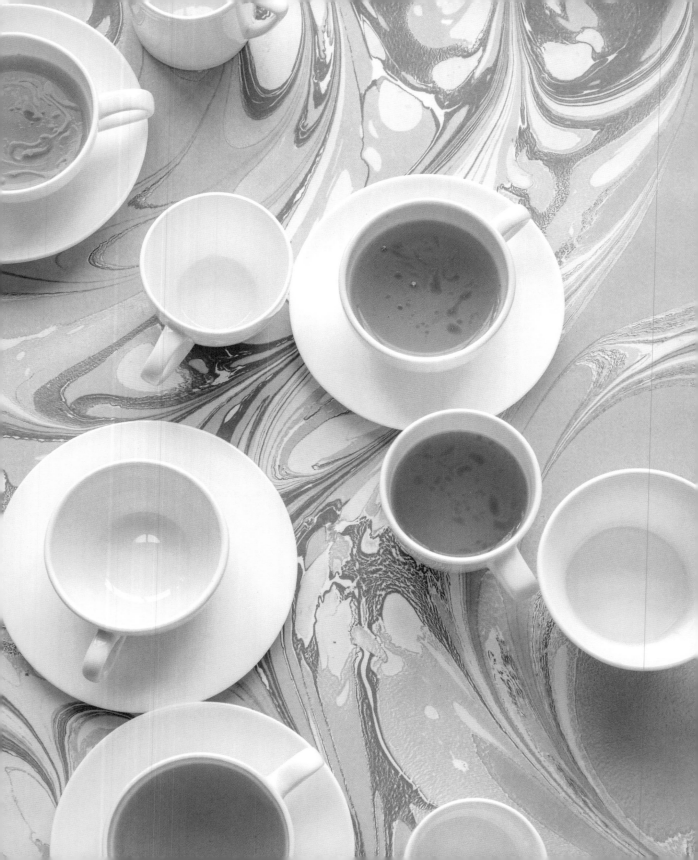

WOMEN'S HEALTH CBD INFUSION

Particularly good for the week leading up to your period, this tea can help with blood flow, pain and uterine health.

1 tablespoon dried raspberry leaves
1 tablespoon dried red clover
1 tablespoon dried chamomile flowers
1 teaspoon dried damiana leaves
1 litre/quart hot water (boiled and then cooled for about 2–5 minutes)
¼ teaspoon CBD oil and half a mug of just-boiled water, per serving

1 litre/quart glass mason/kilner jar with a lid

MAKES 3–4 SERVINGS

Combine all the herbs and hot water in the mason/kilner jar. Mix so that the herbs are submerged in the water and place the lid on. Leave to infuse for a minimum of 4 hours or overnight at room temperature.

Strain the infusion and discard the herbs. Pour the liquid into a clean jar, or rinse out and use the same jar again. The infusion will keep at room temperature for 2–3 days or refrigerated for up to 1 week.

Serve the infusion warm by combining half a mug of the infusion with half a mug of just-boiled water. Stir ¼ teaspoon CBD oil into the warm liquid and enjoy.

GREEN VITAMINS & MINERALS CBD INFUSION

///////////////

This is my favourite everyday herbal infusion – simple and chock-full of vitamins and minerals. Nettles bring iron and vitamin C along with anti-inflammatory and pain-relieving properties, while peppermint is a good source of zinc, vitamin A and several B vitamins and it refreshes and soothes. Sometimes I'll add a bit of my other favourite herb – lemon balm – to this one as well.

1 tablespoon dried nettles
2 tablespoons dried peppermint
1 litre/quart hot water
(boiled and then cooled for about 2–5 minutes)
¼ teaspoon CBD oil and half a mug of just-boiled water per serving, to serve

1 litre/quart glass mason/kilner jar with a lid

MAKES 3–4 SERVINGS

Combine all the herbs and hot water in the mason/kilner jar. Mix so that the herbs are submerged in the water and place the lid on. Leave to infuse for a minimum of 4 hours or overnight at room temperature.

Strain the infusion and discard the herbs. Pour the liquid into a clean jar, or rinse out and use the same jar again. The infusion will keep at room temperature for 2–3 days or refrigerated for up to 1 week.

Serve the infusion warm by combining half a mug of the infusion with half a mug of just-boiled water. Stir ¼ teaspoon CBD oil into the warm liquid and enjoy.

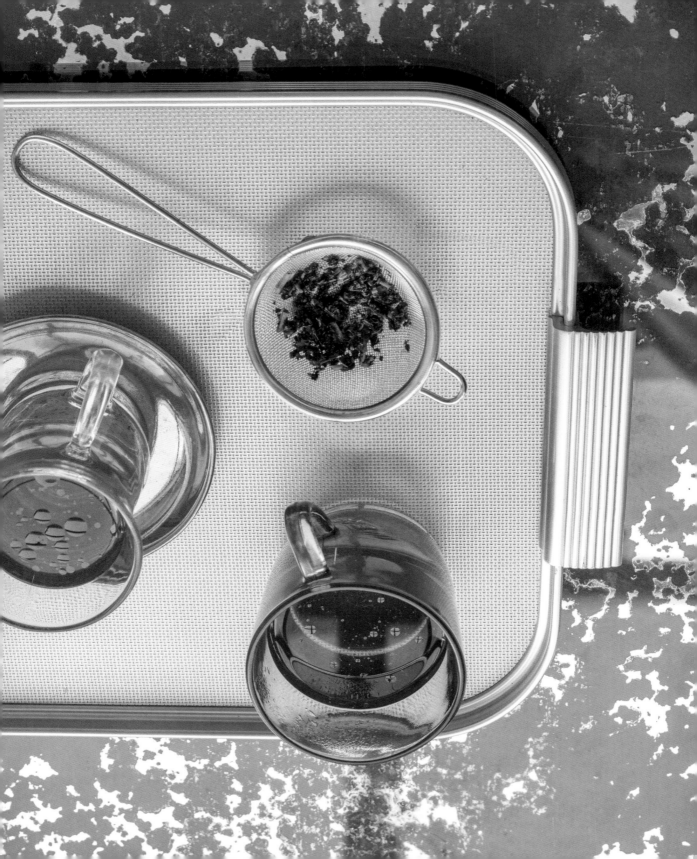

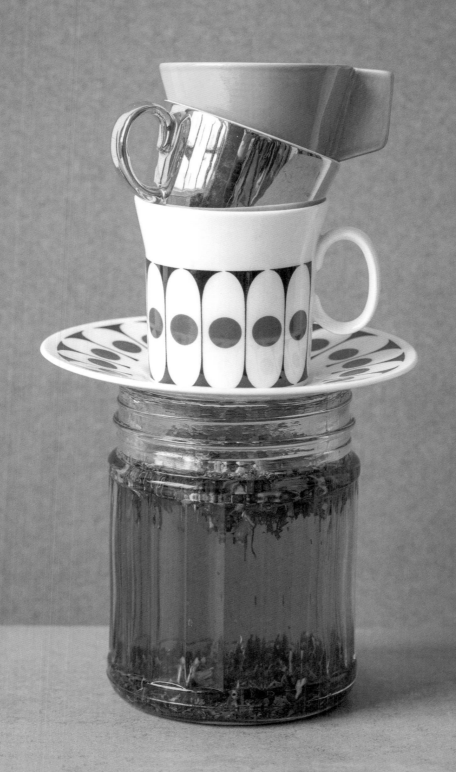

DIGESTION
CBD INFUSION

//////////////

This powerful combination uses stimulating ginger and fennel to aid the digestion process, and chamomile and lemon balm to quell any stress your system might be under. Stress is often an underlying cause of bad digestion and learning to calm our minds and bodies can have a big impact.

MAKES 3–4 SERVINGS

2.5-cm/1-inch piece of fresh ginger, peeled and thinly sliced
1 tablespoon fennel seeds
1 tablespoon dried chamomile flowers
1 tablespoon dried lemon balm leaves
1 litre/quart hot water (boiled and then cooled for about 2–5 minutes)
¾ teaspoon CBD oil and half a mug of just-boiled water per serving, to serve
1 litre/quart glass mason/kilner jar with a lid

Combine the ginger, all the herbs and hot water in the mason/kilner jar. Mix so that the ginger and herbs are submerged in the water and place the lid on. Leave to infuse for a minimum of 4 hours or overnight at room temperature. Strain the infusion and discard the ginger and herbs. Pour the liquid into a clean jar, or rinse out and use the same jar again. The infusion will keep at room temperature for 2–3 days or refrigerated for up to 1 week.

Serve the infusion warm by combining half a mug of the infusion with half a mug of just-boiled water. Stir ¾ teaspoon CBD oil into the warm liquid and enjoy.

IMMUNITY CBD INFUSION

///////////

When you feel a cold coming on, reach for this combo.
You can add a little fresh, finely grated ginger to this
one too, if you'd like.

2 tablespoons dried elderberries
1 tablespoon dried echinacea
freshly squeezed juice of 1 small
   lemon
1 tablespoon honey (optional)
1 litre/quart hot water
   (boiled and then cooled for
   about 2–5 minutes)
¼ teaspoon CBD oil and half
   a mug of just-boiled water
   per serving, to serve

*1 litre/quart glass mason jar
with a lid*

MAKES 3–4 SERVINGS

Combine all the herbs and hot water in the
mason/kilner jar. Mix so that the herbs are
submerged in the water and place the lid on.
Leave to infuse for a minimum of 4 hours or
overnight at room temperature.

Strain the infusion and discard the herbs.
Stir in the lemon juice and honey (if using). Pour
the liquid into a clean jar, or rinse out and use
the same jar again. The infusion will keep at
room temperature for 2–3 days or refrigerated
for up to 1 week.

Serve the infusion warm by combining half
a mug of the infusion with half a mug of just-
boiled water. Stir ¼ teaspoon CBD oil into the
warm liquid and enjoy.

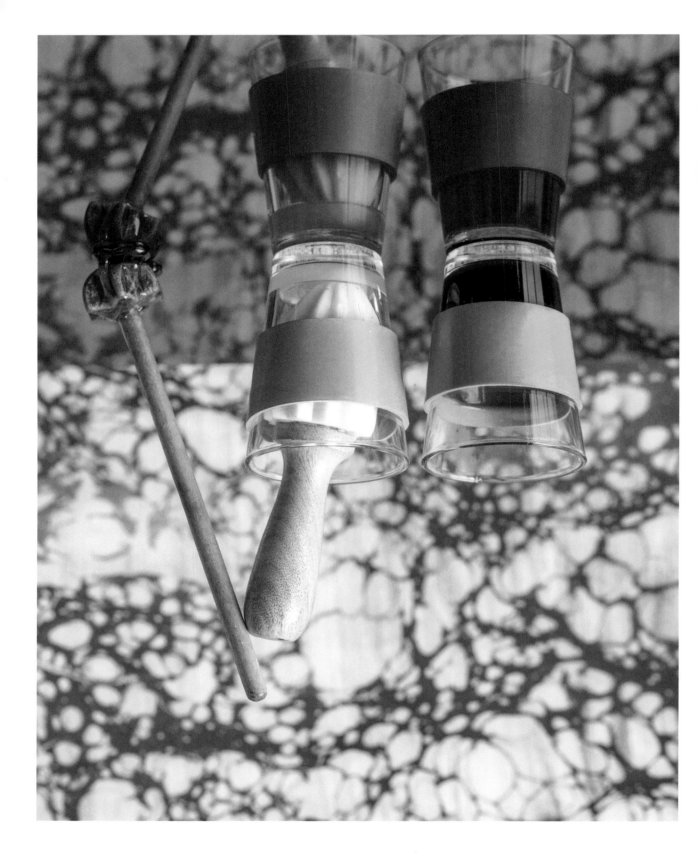

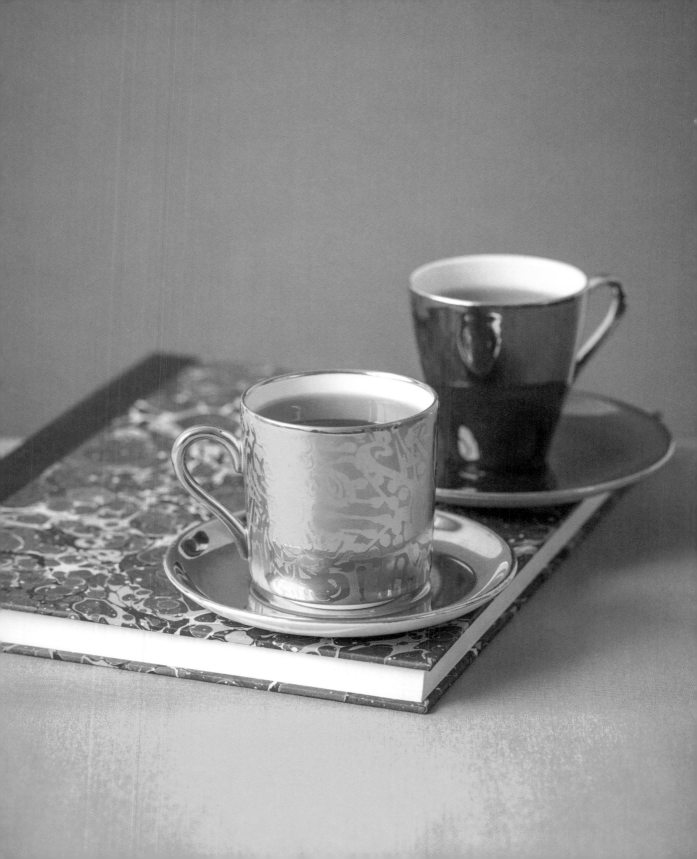

BRAIN BOOSTER CBD INFUSION

These herbs aid both blood flow and brain function, helping to increase focus and alleviate stressors.

1 tablespoon oat straw
1 tablespoon dried peppermint
½ tablespoon gotu kola
½ tablespoon tulsi
1 litre/quart hot water
 (boiled and then cooled for
 about 2–5 minutes)
¼ teaspoon CBD oil and half
 a mug of just-boiled water
 per serving, to serve

*1 litre/quart glass mason jar
with a lid*

MAKES 3–4 SERVINGS

Combine all the herbs and hot water in the mason/kilner jar. Mix so that the herbs are submerged in the water and place the lid on. Leave to infuse for a minimum of 4 hours or overnight at room temperature.

Strain the infusion and discard the herbs. Pour the liquid into a clean jar, or rinse out and use the same jar again. The infusion will keep at room temperature for 2–3 days or refrigerated for up to 1 week.

Serve the infusion warm by combining half a mug of the infusion with half a mug of just-boiled water. Stir ¼ teaspoon CBD oil into the warm liquid and enjoy.

HEART OPENER CBD INFUSION

///////////////

Hibiscus infusions are some of my favourites. They're delightfully tart in flavour and become the most beautiful magenta colour as the ingredients infuse. This one combines rose petals and chamomile flowers along with agave syrup, lemon and CBD oil, for a visually pretty, calming blend.

2 tablespoons dried hibiscus flowers
2 tablespoons dried chamomile flowers
3 tablespoons dried food grade rose petals
1 litre/quart hot water (boiled and then slightly cooled for about 2–5 minutes)

TO SERVE
2 tablespoons freshly squeezed lemon juice
1 tablespoon agave syrup (optional)
¼–½ teaspoon CBD oil per serving, to serve

large sterilized litre/quart jar with a lid

MAKES 3–4 SERVINGS

Combine all the dried flowers and petals with the hot water in the jar. Mix so that they are submerged in the water and place the lid on the jar. Leave to infuse for a minimum of 4 hours or overnight at room temperature.

Strain the infusion and discard the flowers. Pour the mixture back into a clean jar, or rinse out and use the same jar again. Add the lemon juice, agave syrup (if using) and CBD oil. Put the lid back on the jar and shake to combine the ingredients.

Add a little extra hot water and serve warm in a mug, or serve the infusion cold over ice in a tall glass. The infusion will keep well at room temperature or in the refrigerator for up to 3 days.

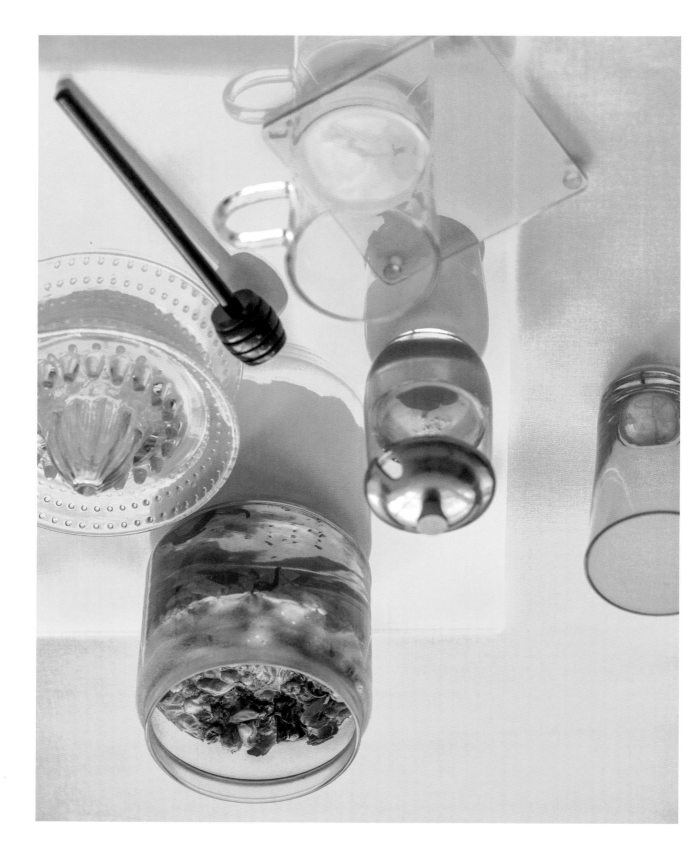

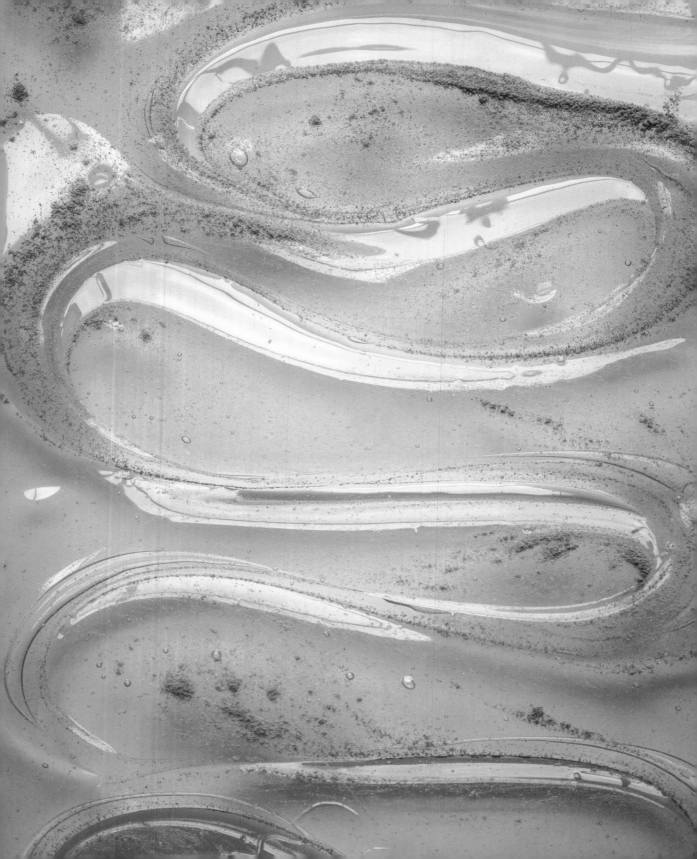

Soothe aches and pains or stressed-out skin with these home-made anti-inflammatory beauty products.

SKINCARE

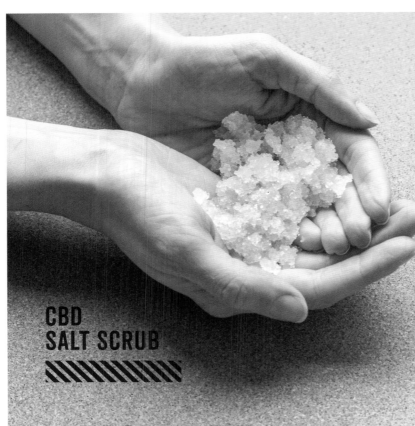

CBD
SALT SCRUB

Exfoliating, moisturizing and pain-relieving, this scrub
is easily made and can be used two to three times a week.
I love to add lavender for its calming qualities, but you
can use one of your own favourite essential oils – just
be careful of using citrus oils in the morning, as they can
make your skin more sensitive to the sun.

200 g/1 cup Epsom salts
60 ml/¼ cup avocado oil or sweet
   almond oil
2 teaspoons CBD oil
10–15 drops of lavender essential
   oil or other essential oil of your
   choice

*250 ml/1 cup capacity shallow jar
with a lid*

MAKES APPROX. 200 G/1 CUP

Place the salt in the jar and pour over the
avocado or sweet almond oil, CBD oil and
lavender essential oil (or essential oil of your
choice). Give it a stir to combine everything
and cover with the lid.

Stored in the sealed jar in your bathroom,
this amount of scrub should last you about
1 month, but will keep for 2–3 months.

To use Take a palm-full of the scrub in the
shower and massage into wet skin, focusing on
any sore or dry areas. Rinse off with warm water.

CBD ANTI-INFLAMMATORY FACE MASK

Honey is a powerful yet gentle face cleanser because it's both antimicrobial and moisturizing. When combined with anti-inflammatory CBD oil and cinnamon (which also acts as a mild exfoliant), this mask will reduce blemishes and redness in a gentle way, leaving your skin softer, less inflamed and more even in tone.

1 teaspoon manuka honey
¼ teaspoon CBD oil
⅛ teaspoon ground cinnamon

MAKES 1 MASK

In a small bowl, mix the three ingredients together.

To use Apply to a clean face in a thin layer (avoiding contact with the eyes) and leave on the skin for at least 15 minutes or up to 1 hour. Rinse the mask off with warm water and moisturize as normal.

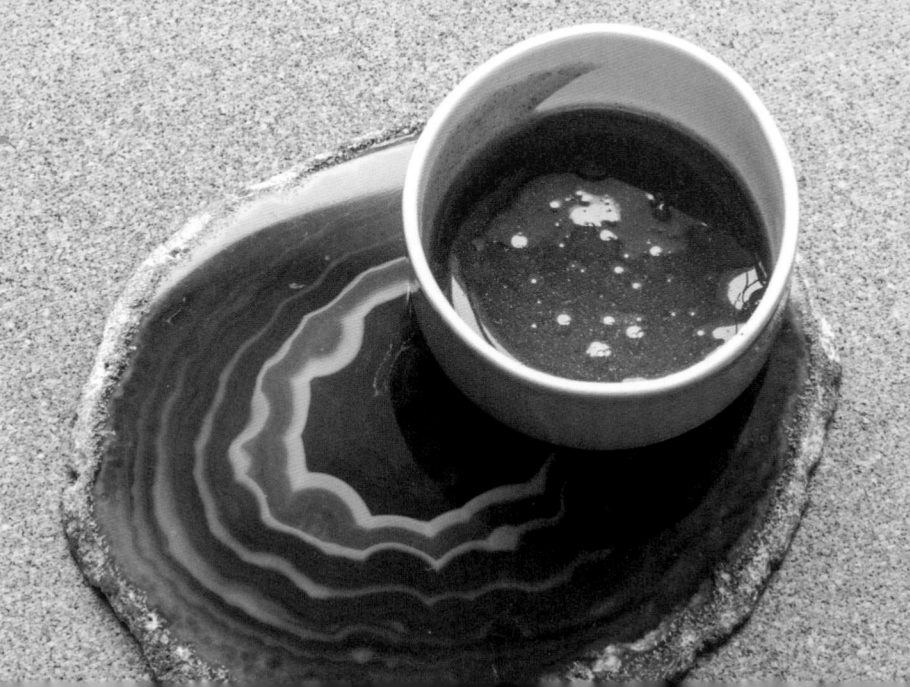

CBD NIGHT-TIME MOISTURIZING FACE OIL

///////////

Sweet orange essential oil adds a natural hit of vitamin C, which helps to even out and brighten skin tone – but don't use it on your face during the day because it can make your skin more sensitive to sunlight. The rosehip and jojoba oils moisturize and bring skin-supportive vitamin E, while the CBD does its anti-inflammatory thing.

2 tablespoons rosehip oil
2 tablespoons jojoba oil
2 teaspoons CBD oil
10 drops sweet orange essential oil

small, airtight dark glass bottle, ideally with a glass dropper

MAKES 70 G/2½ OZ.

Combine the ingredients in the glass bottle and shake vigorously to combine everything.

Stored in a cool place out of direct sunlight, the face oil should keep for 2–3 months in the airtight dark glass bottle.

To use After cleansing and toning in the evening, apply 2–3 drops to the face, gently massaging into the skin and avoiding contact with your eyes.

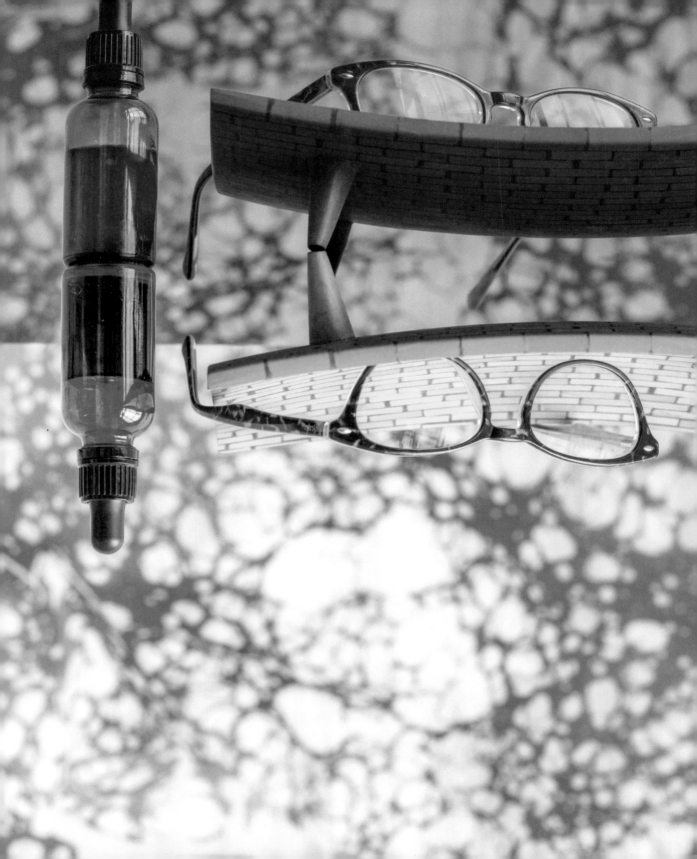

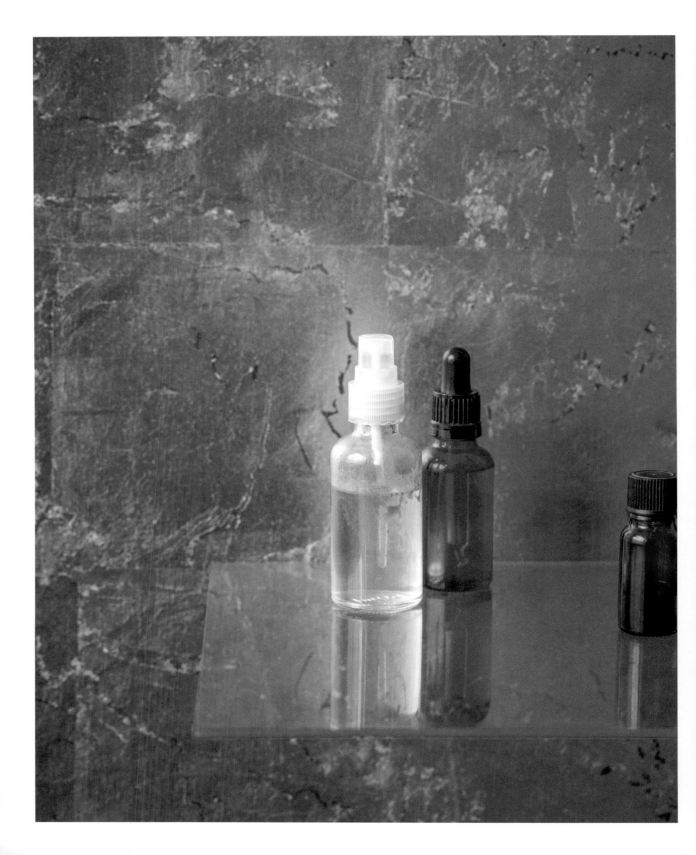

CBD FACIAL
TONER

A good toner can both hydrate and tighten pores while helping your moisturizer work better – especially if you're using a facial oil (like the CBD Night-time Moisturizing Face Oil on page 114).

60 ml/¼ cup rosewater
1 tablespoon witch hazel
1 teaspoon pure aloe vera juice
1 teaspoon CBD oil

small, airtight glass spray bottle

MAKES 90 ML/3 OZ.

Combine the ingredients in your small spray bottle. Shake to combine everything.

Stored in a cool place out of direct sunlight, the toner should keep for 2–3 months in the airtight bottle.

To use Shake before using and spritz 1–3 sprays onto your face after cleansing and before moisturizing. Avoid contact with your eyes.

CBD BODY BUTTER

//////////////

The combination of magnesium oil, CBD oil and clary sage or lavender essential oil make this the ultimate pain-relieving balm. This body butter is great for any kind of muscle ache, but especially for period cramps – when they hit, simply rub this body butter into the lower abdomen. Apply before using a hot water bottle and you'll have a natural pain reliever that works super fast.

100 g/½ cup coconut oil
100 g/½ cup raw cocoa butter, roughly chopped
3 tablespoons magnesium oil
2–3 teaspoons CBD oil
15 drops clary sage or lavender essential oil

airtight container

MAKES ABOUT 235 G/ GENEROUS 1 CUP

In a small saucepan over a low heat, melt the coconut oil and cocoa butter. Once liquid, remove from the heat and stir in the magnesium oil, CBD oil and clary sage or lavender essential oil. Transfer to a bowl and let the mixture cool and firm back up to the texture of butter (it may need refrigerating for 15–20 minutes if your home is warm).

Using a hand-held mixer or electric whisk, whip the mixture for about 1–2 minutes until you have a fluffy body butter. Transfer to an airtight container.

Kept in a cool place out of direct sunlight, the body butter should keep for 2–3 months in the airtight container.

To use Rub in to any skin anywhere you're experiencing aches and pains.

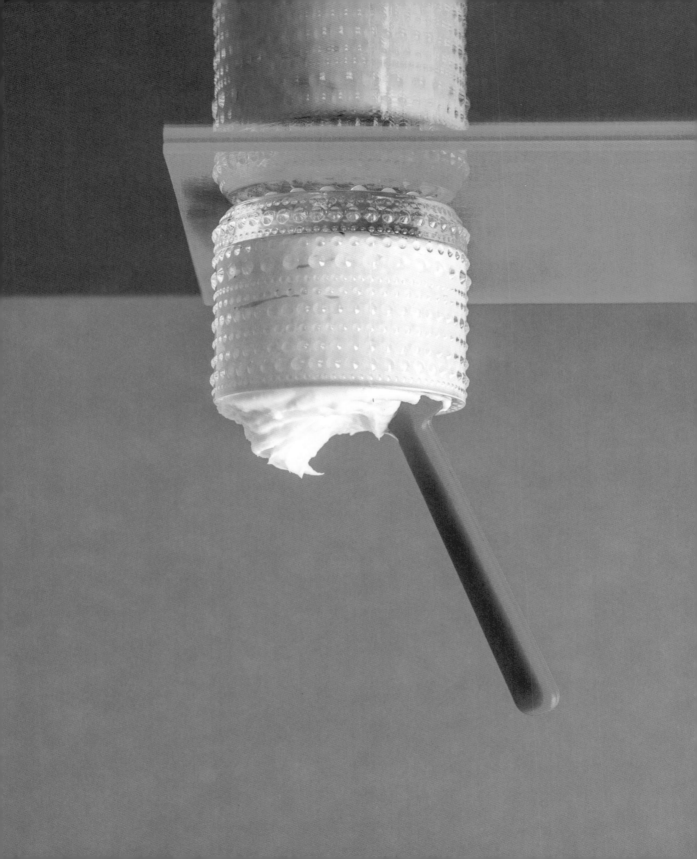

YOUR CBD SCHEDULE

The time of day you choose to take CBD is entirely up to you. Some people prefer it first thing in the morning, especially if they have a stressful day ahead, while others opt for an evening dose to help them relax in preparation for sleep. There's also a case for midday consumption to calm the mind in order to power through the rest of a packed afternoon. You can choose to take it once a day, twice or morning, noon and night – the right dosage and amount to take, as well as the timing of it, is completely up to you. As always, try things out and see how your body responds. If it helps, keep doing it and if it doesn't sit well, try something else. To help you decide on the right routine:

1. Identify why you're taking CBD, which should tell you when you might want to feel its effects most.

2. Identify the right amount for you. Remember to start small and spread the amount over the course of the day to see what feels best.

3. Switch it up and try out a few variations until you find what works best.

MORNING

Taking CBD in the morning is great for:
- Aches and pains/inflammation
- Anxiety or stress about the day ahead
- Period cramps or PMS
- Low mood

If you find that taking CBD in the morning can either make you drowsy or a little too relaxed, try a smaller amount. That being said, a morning dose isn't for everyone, and I have personally only taken it in the mornings when I'm dealing with anxiety on a regular basis or in the lead-up to my period.

Making CBD a part of a morning ritual can include mindfully making and enjoying a latte or breakfast with it. You can also take it in combination with some meditating or gentle stretching and breathing to get your blood flowing. It's great if you can find a small moment of calm to start the day – even if just for a couple of minutes – to connect to yourself and your body and to calm the mind.

RECOMMENDED CBD RECIPES FOR THE MORNING
- Matcha Latte (see page 18)
- Coffee Tonic (see page 21)
- Chai Latte (see page 22)
- Mango & Ginger Smoothie (see page 30)
- Green Strawberry Smoothie (see page 26)
- Beet Berry Smoothie (see page 26)
- Super-Powered Yogurt Bowl (see page 33)
- Snacking Granola Clusters (see page 34)

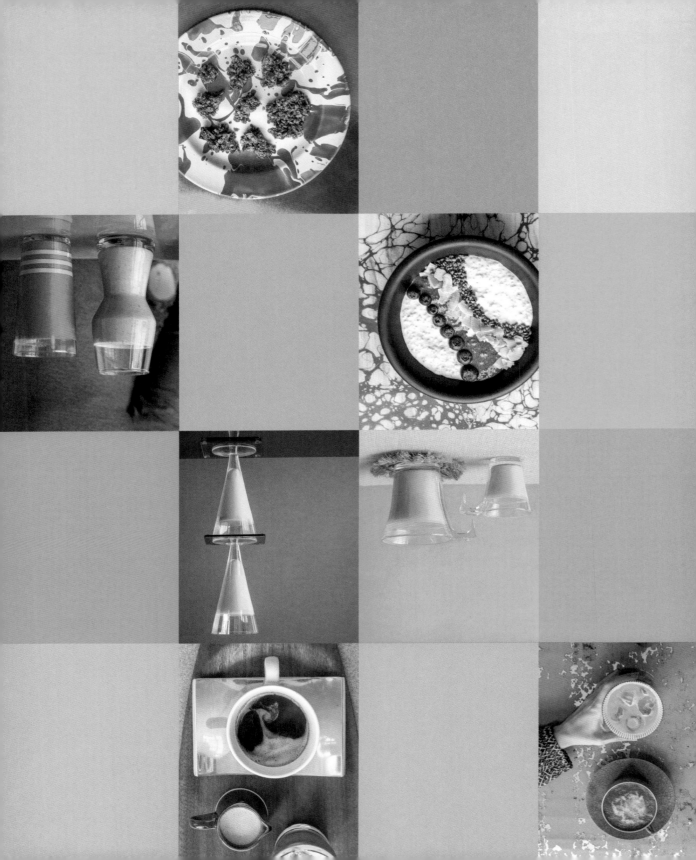

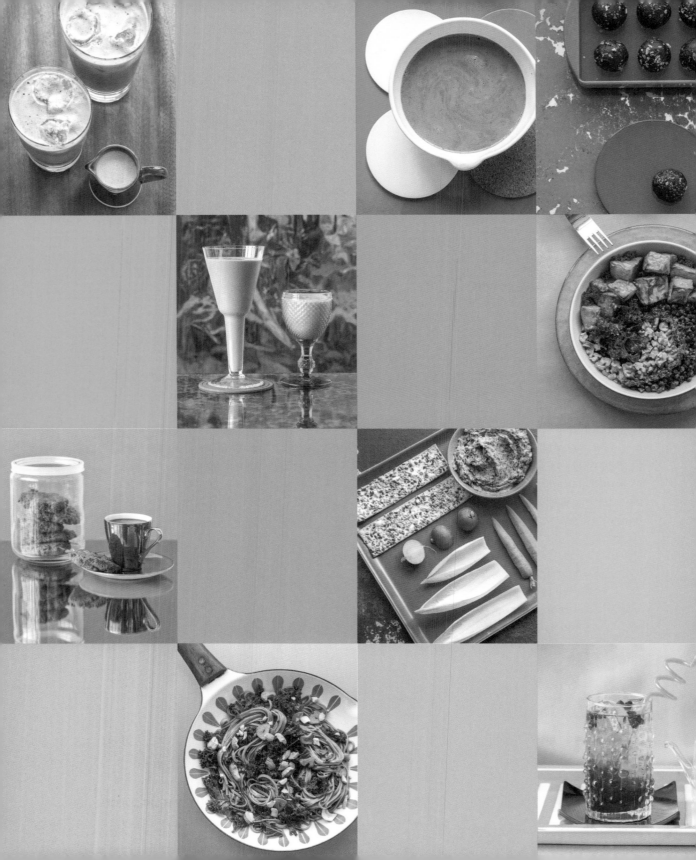

NOON

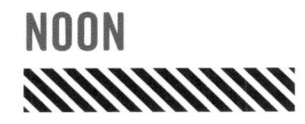

An afternoon serving of CBD can be useful in dealing with:

- Workday stressors
- Post-workout inflammation
- Pain management
- Focus (or lack thereof)

Similarly to taking CBD in the morning, taking it midday might not be perfect for everyone every day, if it makes you a little too relaxed when coupled with that post-lunch slump. Pay attention to what your body needs on any given day and how you might be able to effectively use CBD to help you. Personally it's helped me with afternoon headaches and pairs perfectly with a 5-minute meditation to realign my focus.

Some useful strategies I couple with CBD in the afternoon (if I'm feeling stretched too thin, anxious or unfocused) include taking a quick walk, eating lunch away from screens – with other people and/or outside if possible – and spending a few minutes to just sit and breathe.

RECOMMENDED CBD RECIPES FOR THE AFTERNOON

- Dandelion Iced Coffee Tonic (see page 21)
- Hot Cacao (see page 22)
- Raw Brownie Bites (see page 38)
- Chocolate & Peanut Butter Smoothie (see page 29)
- Pumpkin Choc Chip Cookies (see page 49)
- Herby White Bean & Garlic Dip (see page 73)
- Lentil & Sweet Potato Bowl with Chimichurri (see page 78)
- Soba Noodles, Kale & Cashews with Garlic & Chilli Oil (see page 81)
- Pomegranate & Kombucha Mocktail (see page 93)

NIGHT

CBD in the evening can help with:

- Improving sleep
- Calming that bedtime thought loop
- Relaxing and shutting down the engines
- Reducing inflammation accumulated over the course of the day

I love CBD in the evenings. It's great if you have an overactive brain like so many of us do. You can take it about an hour before sleep to give you a restful night of shut-eye or perhaps in a nightcap to help you unwind from the day.

When I find myself still scatterbrained and wired from the day, I like to take CBD in combination with some phone- and computer-free time. I also turn down any really bright lights in favour of smaller, softer lighting – like the peachy-pink glow from a Himalayan salt lamp or warm candlelight. If I'm Netflixing it, I'll wear my anti-blue light glasses, turn the brightness down on my TV screen and put my phone in another room – multiple screens can be too much that late in the day.

If I'm trying to get to sleep and struggling a little, I'll do the 4-7-8 breathing technique. It's simple: breathe in for 4 counts, hold your breath for 7 counts and slowly breathe out for 8 counts. Repeat as needed. This breathing sequence can help calm the nervous system, slow your heart rate and help you focus on something other than your thoughts – which all help to prepare the body for sleep.

RECOMMENDED CBD RECIPES FOR NIGHT-TIME

- Turmeric Latte (see page 16)
- Rose Latte (see page 17)
- Pistachio & Tahini Bites (see page 42)
- Chocolate Pudding (see page 54)
- Tomato & Butternut Soup with Pesto (see page 66)
- Roasted Potato & Tomato Bake with Olive Oil, Shallot & Lemon Dressing (see page 77)
- Ginger & Lime Mocktail (see page 92)
- Grapefruit & Rose Mocktail (see page 92)
- Elderflower Spritz (see page 89)
- Simple Margarita (see page 89)

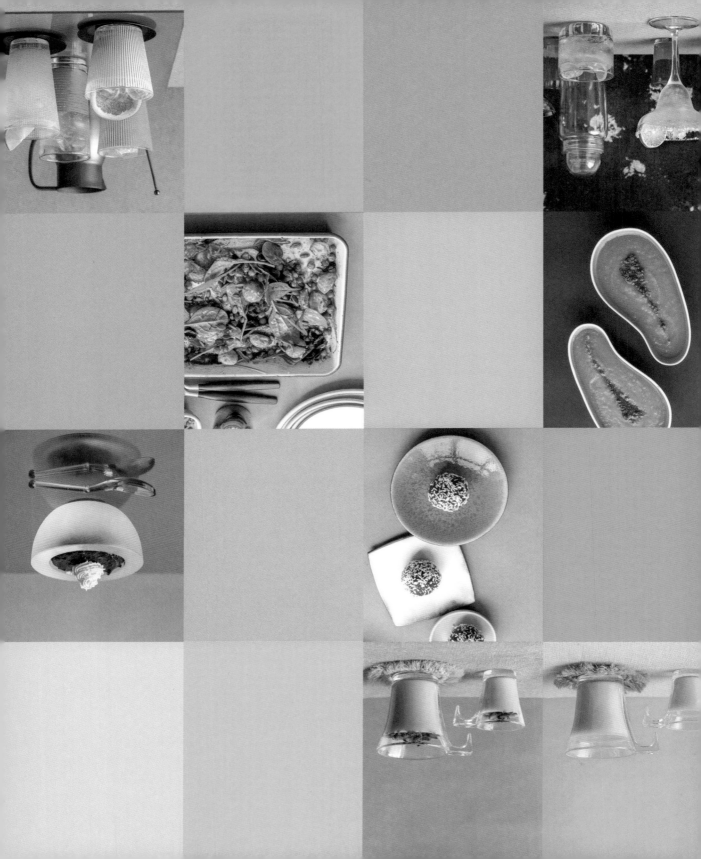

INDEX

A

anti-anxiety CBD infusion 96
anti-inflammatory face mask, CBD 113
anxiety 6, 8
avocados: CBD avocado toast 70
CBD chocolate pudding 54

B

bake, roasted potato & tomato 77
bananas: CBD banana & cinnamon smoothie 29
CBD raspberry & banana nice cream 50
bark, CBD sea salt & cacao nib chocolate 57
basil: CBD pesto 66
beans: CBD herby white bean & garlic dip 73
beetroot/beets: CBD beet berry smoothie 26
CBD beetroot latte 18
berries: CBD beet berry smoothie 26
CBD berry gummies 63
blackberries: CBD gin & blackberry bramble 86
body butter, CBD 118
brain booster CBD infusion 107
bread: CBD avocado toast 70
brownie bites, CBD raw 38
butternut squash: tomato & butternut soup 66

C

cacao: CBD chocolate & peanut butter smoothie 29
CBD chocolate pudding 54
CBD hot cacao 22
CBD mint chocolate bites 45
CBD raw brownie bites 38
CBD reishi cacao cashew fudgesicles 53
CBD sea salt & cacao nib chocolate bark 57
caramels, CBD date 58
cashews: CBD reishi cacao cashew fudgesicles 53
soba noodles, kale & cashews 81
CBD (cannabidiol) oil: benefits of 6-9
how much to take 11
how to cook with 12
how to take it 10
reasons to cook with 12
vs hemp seed oil 10
vs THC 9-10
what to look for when buying 10-11
where to buy 10
chai latte, CBD 22
chickpea/gram flour: green chickpea CBD pancakes 82
chickpeas: grilled lettuce, chickpea & radish salad 74
chimichurri, CBD 78
chocolate: CBD

chocolate & peanut butter smoothie 29
CBD chocolate pudding 54
CBD date caramels 58
CBD hot cacao 22
CBD mint chocolate bites 45
CBD pumpkin choc chip cookies 49
CBD raw brownie bites 38
CBD raw oatmeal cookie bites 46
CBD reishi cacao cashew fudgesicles 53
CBD sea salt & cacao nib chocolate bark 57
cocktails 86-9
coconut: CBD coconut & pecan bites 41
coconut milk: CBD beet berry smoothie 26
CBD beetroot latte 18
CBD chocolate & peanut butter smoothie 29
CBD matcha latte 18
coffee: CBD coffee tonic 21
cookie bites, CBD raw oatmeal 46
cookies, CBD pumpkin choc chip 49
courgettes: CBD leek & courgette soup 69

D

dandelion tea: CBD dandelion iced coffee tonic 21
dates: CBD coconut & pecan bites 41

CBD date caramels 58
CBD mint chocolate bites 45
CBD raw brownie bites 38
depression 8
digestion CBD infusion 103
dip, CBD herby white bean & garlic 73

E

elderflower liqueur: CBD elderflower spritz 89
endocannabinoid system 8

F

face mask, CBD anti-inflammatory 113
face oil, CBD night-time moisturizing 114
facial toner, CBD 117
fudgesicles, CBD reishi cacao cashew 53

G

gin: CBD gin & blackberry bramble 86
CBD Tom Collins 86
ginger: CBD ginger & lime mocktail 92
CBD mango & ginger smoothie 30
granola clusters, CBD snacking 34
grapefruit: CBD grapefruit & rose mocktail 92
gummies: CBD berry gummies 63
CBD mango gummies 62

H
heart opener CBD infusion 108
hemp 6, 9
hemp seed oil, vs CBD oil 10
herbs: CBD chimichurri 78
    CBD herby white bean & garlic dip 73

I
immunity CBD infusion 104
infusions 96–109

K
kale: lentil sweet potato bowl 78
    soba noodles, kale & cashews with CBD garlic & chilli oil 81
kombucha: CBD pomegranate & kombucha mocktail 91

L
lattes 16–22
leeks: CBD leek & courgette soup 69
lentil sweet potato bowl 78
lettuce: grilled lettuce, chickpea & radish salad 74
limes: CBD ginger & lime mocktail 92

M
mangoes: CBD mango & ginger smoothie 30
    CBD mango gummies 62

margarita, simple CBD 89
marijuana 9, 11
matcha latte, CBD 18
minerals: green vitamins & minerals CBD infusion 100
mocktails 90–2

N
'nice' cream, CBD raspberry & banana 50
night-time moisturizing face oil 114
noodles: soba noodles, kale & cashews with CBD garlic & chilli oil 81

O
oats: CBD raw oatmeal cookie bites 46
    CBD snacking granola clusters 34
    CBD super-powered yogurt bowl 33
oil-based tinctures 10

P
pancakes, green chickpea CBD 82
peanut butter: CBD chocolate & peanut butter smoothie 29
pecans: CBD coconut & pecan bites 41
pesto, CBD 66
phytocannabinoids 8, 9, 11
pineapple: CBD pineapple & mint smoothie 31
pistachios: CBD

pistachio & tahini bites 42
pomegranate juice: CBD pomegranate & kombucha mocktail 91
potatoes: roasted potato & tomato bake 77
Prosecco: CBD elderflower spritz 89
pumpkin: CBD pumpkin choc chip cookies 49

R
radishes: grilled lettuce, chickpea & radish salad 74
raspberries: CBD raspberry & banana nice cream 50
reishi mushroom powder: CBD reishi cacao cashew fudgesicles 53
rosewater: CBD grapefruit & rose mocktail 92
    CBD rose latte 17

S
salad, grilled lettuce, chickpea & radish 74
salt scrub, CBD 112
schedule, CBD 120–4
skincare 110–19
sleep 8
smoothies 26–31
soups: CBD leek & courgette soup 69
    tomato & butternut soup with CBD pesto 66
strawberries: CBD green

strawberry smoothie 26
sweet potatoes: lentil sweet potato bowl 78

T
tahini: CBD pistachio & tahini bites 42
tequila: simple CBD margarita 89
THC (tetrahydrocannabinol) 9–10
tinctures, oil-based 10
Tom Collins, CBD 86
tomatoes: roasted potato & tomato bake 77
    tomato & butternut soup 66
tonics: CBD coffee tonic 21
    CBD dandelion iced coffee tonic 21
turmeric latte, CBD 16

V
vitamins: green vitamins & minerals CBD infusion 100

W
walnuts: CBD snacking granola clusters 34
    lentil sweet potato bowl 78
watermelon mocktail, CBD 90
women's health CBD infusion 99

Y
yogurt: CBD super-powered yogurt bowl 33

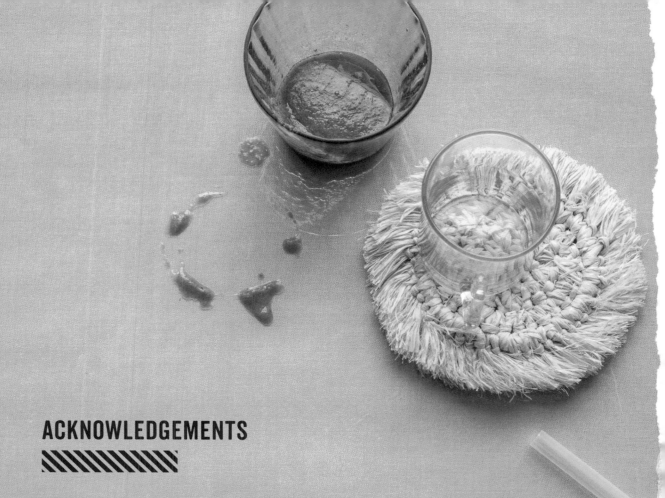

ACKNOWLEDGEMENTS
////////////////////

Thank you to Cindy Richards and Alice Sambrook for getting excited about this book. As always, thank you to my agent Sharon Bowers for miraculously making things happen. Thanks to Megan Smith, Maud Eden, Alexander Breeze and Clare Winfield for bringing my recipes to life in new and beautiful ways. And to Fabian, my biggest supporter with the best accent, thank you.